Sports
Medicine
for
Coaches
and
Trainers

Edward J. Shahady, M.D.

Michael J. Petrizzi, M.D.

SPORTS MEDICINE for Coaches and Trainers

Second Edition

The University of

North Carolina Press

Chapel Hill and London

First edition published in 1988.

The paper in this book meets the guidelines for permanence
and durability of the Committee on Production Guidelines
for Book Longevity of the Council on Library Resources.
95 94 93 92 91   5 4 3 2 1

Library of Congress Cataloging-in-Publication Data

Shahady, Edward J.
    Sports medicine for coaches and trainers / Edward J.
Shahady, Michael J. Petrizzi.—2nd ed.
        p.   cm.
    ISBN 0-8078-1991-3 (cloth : alk. paper).—
ISBN 0-8078-4331-8 (pbk. : alk. paper)
    1. Sports medicine.   2. Athletes—Wounds and
injuries.   3. Coaches (Athletics)   I. Petrizzi, Michael J.
II. Title.
RC1210.S52   1991
617.1'027—dc20   91-2604
                                                         CIP

Illustrations by Harold Rydberg

To my best friend and wife, Sandra, for her encouragement and beautiful smile.

    To my children, Mary, John, Tom, Lisa, Ed, and
Bill. Their participation in sports from Little League
through college provided me an excellent reason
to become knowledgeable about sports medicine.—Ed Shahady

To my wife, Kathy, for all her love, patience, and
understanding.

    To my family and Kathy's family for all their
support.—Mike Petrizzi

To each other—mutual respect and stimulation
gave us the energy to dream, plan, and complete
this book.

Contents

Contributors

Affiliations listed below indicate the status of the contributors at the time the first edition of this book was written.

Salli Benedict, M.P.H.
Health Educator
Department of Family Medicine
University of North Carolina
Chapel Hill, North Carolina

John E. Blake, A.T.C.
Athletic Trainer
Southern High School
Durham, North Carolina

Mary G. Broos, M.S.
Head Athletic Trainer
Guilford College
Greensboro, North Carolina

Beverly Brown, M.A.T., A.T.C.
Head Trainer
Chapel Hill High School
Chapel Hill, North Carolina

Peter R. Coleman, M.D.
Former Family Practice Resident
University of North Carolina
Chapel Hill, North Carolina

Michael J. DeBevec, M.D.
Former Bush Sports Medicine Fellow
University of North Carolina
Chapel Hill, North Carolina

Joseph L. DeWalt, M.D.
Director, Sports Medicine
Team Physician
University of North Carolina
Chapel Hill, North Carolina

Anthony J. Geraci, Jr., M.D.
Former Family Practice Resident
University of North Carolina
Chapel Hill, North Carolina

Donald Ives, M.D.
Former Medical Student
University of North Carolina
Chapel Hill, North Carolina

Timothy J. Ives, Pharm.D.
Assistant Professor, School of Pharmacy
University of North Carolina
Chapel Hill, North Carolina

Richard L. Knox
Associate Executive Director
North Carolina High School Athletic Association
Chapel Hill, North Carolina

John C. LaLonde, M.D.
Team Physician
Guilford College
Greensboro, North Carolina

Robbie H. Lester, M.Ed., A.T.C.
Chief Consultant, Sports Medicine Program
Department of Public Instruction
Raleigh, North Carolina

J. Thomas Newton, M.D.
Family Physician
Clinton Medical Clinic
Clinton, North Carolina

Michael J. Petrizzi, M.D.
Assistant Professor of Family Practice
Medical College of Virginia
Virginia Commonwealth University
Richmond, Virginia

Edward J. Shahady, M.D.
Professor of Family Medicine
University of North Carolina
Chapel Hill, North Carolina

Thomas D. Shahady, M.S.P.H.
Doctoral Student
North Carolina State University
Raleigh, North Carolina

Teresa M. Shields, M.D.
Former Family Practice Resident
University of North Carolina
Chapel Hill, North Carolina

Gregory H. Tuttle, M.D.
Family Physician, Assistant Team Physician
University of North Carolina
Chapel Hill, North Carolina

Stanley R. Watson, M.D.
Family Practice Resident
University of North Carolina
Chapel Hill, North Carolina

Thomas J. Zuber, M.D.
Team Physician
South Johnson High School
Benson, North Carolina

Preface

The second edition of this book has benefited from the generous feedback we have received from the first edition. More than two hundred coaches and trainers who used that first edition provided formal written evaluations for our consideration. Their suggestions helped shape the changes incorporated into the second edition.

The first edition used suggestions obtained from coaches and trainers through questionnaires and group interviews. In addition, an advisory committee composed of coaches, trainers, school administrators, parents, and team physicians provided excellent guidance for that first effort.

We hope this new, revised edition will meet the needs of all those who gave us clear and valuable suggestions as well as any others who use the book. We hope to continue to revise the book and would value any suggestions for future editions.

Acknowledgments

We would like to extend our thanks to the following people for their special help in making this book a reality:

Lance Cole, our editorial assistant, for his tireless efforts in translating medical jargon into English. His drive for excellence, patience, and command of the English language form the book's backbone;

Harold Rydberg, for preparing the illustrations for the book, including sixteen new ones for this second edition;

Dick Knox (North Carolina High School Athletic Association), for his encouragement and invaluable guidance;

Robbie Lester (North Carolina Department of Public Instruction), for his insight, enthusiasm, and talent for getting us to the next step;

Bev Brown, the trainer at Chapel Hill High School, for teaching us how to take care of injuries and demonstrating the high-quality care that can be given by trainers;

Coach Bill Hodgin and his fellow coaches at Chapel Hill High School, living examples of coaches who care about their athletes' development not just as players but as people;

Stan Watson, who as a fourth-year medical student helped with research and provided enthusiastic support and advice on many aspects of the book, and who also wrote two chapters;

The student athletes at Chapel Hill High School, who allowed us to care for them while teaching us that athletes are unique individuals who need and deserve the best possible care;

The family practice residents at North Carolina Memorial Hospital, who helped with the care of athletes, especially Mark Guerra and David Jones, who are now in private practice and continue to act as team physicians;

Doctors Joe DeWalt, Tim Taft, and Greg Tuttle and trainers Skip Hunter, Dan Hooker, Bob Smodick, and Mark Davis from the Sports Medicine Program at the University of North Carolina. They shared with us not only their knowledge of sports medicine but also their understanding of how to use that knowledge. Joe DeWalt's understanding of the mechanisms of injuries, coupled with his unique ability to teach patients, students, and colleagues, served as a strong inspiration for the writing of this book;

The Department of Family Medicine at the University of North Carolina, for providing many of the needed resources for publishing this guidebook. Our special thanks to Ruth Williams and Shirley Leighton for their expertise and kindness;

Our advisory committee, for offering outstanding recommendations that helped shape the content of this book;

The many coaches and trainers who completed our questionnaires concerning the content and style of the book. We sincerely hope that we have produced the book you requested;

The physicians and staff at Hanover Family Physicians, for their help in the midnight hours;

The Kate B. Reynolds Foundation, for providing the funds for the first edition.

How to Use This Book

The book is divided into four sections. Section I covers general principles of diagnosis and treatment. This section should be read first because it helps prepare you for the chapters on specific injuries. The section begins by introducing you to some of the terms used in talking about injuries and anatomy. Succeeding chapters describe how to examine the athlete and obtain information about an injury and cover basic principles of treatment such as the use of ice, taping, exercises, stretching, and medications.

Section II begins with a guide to the rapid diagnosis of injuries. This guide allows you to arrive at a quick diagnosis based on the location of the pain, the athlete's symptoms, or the type of injury. The guide is oversimplified, but it may speed up your search for the answer to your athlete's problem.

The rest of Section II, which forms the bulk of the book, focuses on common injuries to specific areas of the body. These chapters will not describe every injury that might occur, but they will probably cover 90 percent of what you are likely to see. Each chapter catalogs the more common injuries to a specific body part. A general description of the injury is followed by a list of symptoms the athlete will display, an explanation of the exam you will need to conduct, and instructions for treatment and prevention of the injury. Many of these chapters end with a set of exercises that can be used to prevent or rehabilitate injuries of that particular body part. You may want to make copies of these exercises to give to your athletes.

The last two sections of the book are not dependent on the first two and therefore can be read out of sequence. Section III covers health problems not related to injury, including skin diseases, heat illness, and medical problems such as high blood pressure and sugar diabetes. Proper nutrition and the unique problems of female athletes are also covered in this section.

Section IV reviews some administrative issues that face all coaches and trainers, for example, developing and equipping the training room and conducting and evaluating preparticipation exams. It also provides some insight into the perspectives of parents and athletes.

Section 1

General
Principles of
Diagnosis and
Treatment

Edward J. Shahady

The Language of Injury

Athletes refer to injuries in terms of the symptoms that keep them from participating, such as pain, a limp, or discomfort. Using symptoms as a beginning, the person trying to make a diagnosis must place the injury into some type of category or define it so that it can be treated. Medical language has been created to help us understand the nature and complexity of injuries and to be more precise in communicating the nature of injuries to others. Following are some terms and their definitions that you should find helpful.

Acute and Chronic Injuries

An **acute** injury happens abruptly, often as a result of a direct blow or a sudden and unnatural stress on a particular body part. A **chronic** injury develops over a period of time, usually due to overuse of a body part.

Overuse Injury

This is a type of chronic injury that usually presents itself acutely. As the term implies, the athlete **overuses** a part of the body, as, for example, when a runner increases mileage from 15 to 50 miles a week within a short period of time. This overload stresses the bones, muscles, and tissues, resulting in inflammation and pain. Stress fractures are a form of overuse injury.

Tendon

A **tendon** is the thick band of tissue at the end of a muscle that attaches to the bone.

Ligament

This is a thick band of tissue that connects one bone to another bone across a space known as a joint. The ligament holds the bones together and keeps the joint stable.

Sprain

A **sprain** is an injury to a ligament. When a ligament is torn or stretched, the joint becomes unstable (weak and loose). The knee and ankle are common locations for sprains.

Sprains are classified by degrees:
- **First degree**—a mild tear
- **Second degree**—a moderate tear
- **Third degree**—a complete tear

Second-degree sprains result in partial instability, third-degree sprains in complete instability.

Strain

A **strain** is a tearing of muscle tissue in the main part (belly) of the muscle or tendon. Strains are also classified by degrees:
- **First degree**—a minimal tear
- **Second degree**—a moderate tear
- **Third degree**—a complete tear

Muscle injuries can take up to nine months to heal, depending on the degree of the tear. The quadriceps and hamstring muscles of the upper leg are examples of commonly strained muscles.

Contusion

Contusion is another word for a bruise or black-and-blue spot. Most contusions cause no trouble aside from the initial discomfort, which usually lasts one or two days. Occasionally a contusion leads to a large amount of bleeding inside a muscle, resulting in swelling and discomfort that can last for several days.

Fracture

This is another word for **broken bone**. There are some special types of fractures:
• **Stress fracture**—a tiny break in one area of a bone, rather than one large break
• **Avulsion fracture**—occurs when a fragment of bone is pulled off by a ruptured tendon or ligament
• **Green stick fracture**—occurs when only one side of the bone is broken, like a green stick
• **Growth plate fracture**—a break in the end of a bone where growth occurs

Dislocation

This is the temporary movement of a bone out of its normal position in a joint. In a dislocation the ligaments and tendons are stretched and sometimes torn. Kneecaps, fingers, and shoulders are the most common areas for dislocations.

Inflammation

Swelling, redness, and pain in a joint or muscle are indications that it is **inflamed**. This condition is usually due to the presence of red and white blood cells and fluid. Inflammation normally occurs after an injury but can also be caused by a bacterial infection.

Edema

Edema is another word for swelling.

Hematoma

A **hematoma** results from a direct blow to a muscle that causes a blood vessel to burst internally and produce swelling or a lump in the muscle. This will later become a black-and-blue mark as the blood comes to the surface.

Subluxation

A **subluxation** is similar to a dislocation, but the bone moves back into its socket without any treatment. Some, like shoulder subluxations, can be recurrent.

Atrophy

Atrophy is the loss of muscle mass that results when muscles are not used.

Hypertrophy

This is an increase in muscle mass commonly seen with exercise and weight training.

Medial

Medial refers to the area toward the inner part or center of the body. For example, the medial part of the knee points toward the other knee, in contrast to the lateral part, which points away from the body.

Lateral

Lateral refers to the area toward the outside of the body, away from other body parts.

Superficial

Superficial refers to the outer part of the body in contrast to the deep or inner part. For example, a superficial burn is a minor burn to the outer skin.

Deep

Deep refers to the inner part of the body in contrast to the superficial. For example, a deep thigh bruise would be in the inner part of the thigh muscles.

Edward J. Shahady

Making a Diagnosis

Each chapter in this book dealing with injuries to a particular part or area of the body is arranged to help you provide the best possible care for injured athletes. The first step in providing that care involves determining as accurately as possible what injury has occurred. This is called making a diagnosis. No treatment, immediate or long-term, can begin without some type of diagnosis being made. When an injury occurs, trying to determine its specific nature and severity can often be a complicated task. The process begins with a recognition of symptoms and circumstances associated with the injury, followed by the exam. Making a diagnosis is somewhat like being a detective—you obtain all the information and see how it all fits together.

Approach

Always approach an injured person calmly and try to instill a sense of calm. This will be more difficult in the event of traumatic injuries than of overuse injuries. Traumatic injuries often happen during competition, and the injured athlete, the other players, and the spectators are all anxious as well as curious. Step in and, using a firm but caring voice, take control of the situation. First, let the athlete know who you are. Even if you know the person well, remember that injured athletes are often disoriented and may not be completely aware of who people are or what is hap-

pening around them. Unless the injury appears to be life-threatening, do not be in a hurry. An athlete's pain will usually decrease within a few minutes, at which time you can do a more thorough evaluation. You may need to do a quick assessment to assure yourself that no life-threatening injury, such as a broken neck, has occurred (see Chapter 7, "Head and Neck Injuries").

Symptoms

The first steps toward interpreting an injured athlete's symptoms involve finding out the circumstances surrounding the injury and, if possible, learning something about the athlete's medical history. **The circumstances surrounding an injury are a crucial factor in determining what injury has occurred**. For instance, in the case of a sprained ankle it is important to know how the foot was planted when the sprain occurred in order to determine which ligament has been sprained. If the injury was accompanied by an audible pop or snap, it could indicate a fracture or a torn ligament. You should also determine whether there was contact with another athlete, the playing surface, or the ball. A hyperextended finger (pushed back by a ball or the playing surface) is treated differently than one that is hyperflexed (pushed in) because a different ligament is torn with each injury.

With overuse injuries, knowledge of an athlete's

medical history as well as the circumstances of the injury can be very useful. Find out if the athlete has made any recent changes in such things as shoes, training, or conditioning routines. **Always keep in mind that old injuries lead to new injuries**. An athlete has a three times greater chance of injuring a particular body part if that part has been previously injured. By meticulously digging out the facts about the mechanics and the circumstances surrounding the injury, you can often have a good idea what the diagnosis is before you begin to examine the athlete. Eighty percent of the diagnosis comes from the history.

Examination

The examination of an injured athlete begins with observation. For instance, look for swelling or discoloration. Black-and-blue marks indicate bleeding underneath the skin. Swelling that occurs immediately is due to blood accumulating in the injured area. Swelling that appears later is due to fluid from inflammation. Both of these signs help in determining the severity of an injury. The more swelling and discoloration is present, the more severe the problem. **Palpation** involves touching or feeling the area surrounding the injury or the injury itself. Do this gently! **Although palpation produces some discomfort, try to train your fingers to find the problem sensitively without aggravating the pain**. Pain produces spasm and spasm makes it difficult to perform the exam. If an athlete twisted an ankle while the foot was plantarflexed (foot pointing down), indicating a torn anterior talofibular ligament, you would feel over the area of this ligament to see if pain and swelling were present. Iliotibial band syndrome and hip pointers are other instances in which feeling over a specific area of the anatomy can help you make a diagnosis.

After palpating the area, you will want to do some manipulations that will help confirm the diagnosis. Stressing the knee by putting pressure on the outside to see if it moves more to one side than the other helps to diagnose torn ligaments. Extending the leg against resistance helps to diagnose thigh bruises, and pushing the foot down against resistance helps to diagnose torn calf muscles. There are other tests to help you determine which part of the anatomy has been affected. Have an athlete move the injured body part. Notice if there is decreased movement and function, or if pain is made

worse by one movement as opposed to another. For instance, being unable to completely extend (straighten) the leg when there is a knee injury usually indicates a torn meniscus (cartilage). Elbow pain when shaking hands is a sign of tennis elbow (epicondylitis). Another useful test consists of moving the injured body part and comparing it to its normal counterpart.

Assessing the range of motion is also an important part of the exam. First, you should test **passive range of motion** by moving the joint through its range of motion without any help from the patient. Note any pain or resistance to motion in the joint or body part. Next, have the patient demonstrate **active range of motion** by moving the body part or joint through its normal range of motion. Note any pain or limitation of motion and compare it to your findings from passive range of motion. You may now proceed to **resistive range of motion**, in which the patient attempts to move the joint or body part while you resist the movement. This comparison of range of motion in the passive, active, and resistive phases helps you recognize which muscles or tendons are injured. A good example of this process is an injury to the rotator cuff of the shoulder. Athletes with this type of injury would have difficulty raising their arms above their heads (active range of motion). You would be able to raise their arms above their heads (passive range of motion) as shown in Figure 21 of Chapter 11, and although you would be able to bring their arms up to a level that they could not, pain would be produced by this movement. You would now resist an attempt to elevate the arm above the head as illustrated in Figure 17 of Chapter 11. You would note any difference in strength between the injured arm and the normal one.

After obtaining a thorough history and performing the examination, you should be able to make a diagnosis 95 percent of the time. Naturally, it will take practice and experience to achieve this degree of accuracy, but it is certainly possible. **The diagnosis you make may be exact or you may be able to narrow an injury down to two or three possibilities— which is okay!**

Once you have a diagnosis, it is time to begin treatment. You may want to have an athlete examined by a physician or call your team physician to ask advice. Treatment options are many and include use of medication, heat, ice, stretching, taping, and rehabilitation. The following chapters will discuss these options.

Edward J. Shahady

3

Treatment
of Injuries

The first few hours and days following an athletic injury are extremely important in the treatment process. Minor injuries can cause a major loss of playing time if certain principles are not followed. Three general principles should guide the treatment of all injuries:
• Initial treatment should include **P-R-I-C-E** (Protection, Rest, Ice, Compression, Elevation).
• Prevent stiffness and muscle atrophy.
• Do not let the athlete lose cardiovascular conditioning.

P-R-I-C-E

Protect the injured body part by splinting the joint, covering the wound, or placing the arm in a sling. Injuries are easily aggravated when they are unprotected.

Rest an injured body part for the first 48 hours. During that time, do not allow the athlete to walk or run on an injured knee or ankle or to use sprained wrists or fingers.

Ice an acute injury for 15 to 20 minutes every 2 to 4 hours for the first 48 hours to keep swelling down. The greater the swelling, the greater the disability.

Compression also helps reduce the swelling. A tightly bound Ace wrap is a must. Check the wrap periodically to assure that it is tight enough but not too tight.

Elevation helps control the swelling. The injured part must be raised above the level of the heart to allow blood and fluid to drain away from the site of the injury. More blood and fluid (swelling) at the site of the injury means greater irritation and a longer recovery period.

Using P-R-I-C-E principles helps decrease pain and bleeding as well as removing blood and fluid from the injured site. For example, a well-managed ankle sprain will not be "black and blue" at the ankle two or three days after the injury; instead, the discoloration will appear further up the leg and on other parts of the foot.

Stiffness and Muscle Atrophy

Although it is important to rest injured parts, it is also important to move them if movement does not cause pain. Joints become stiff and muscles lose strength when they are not moved. Ideally, about 24 hours after injury—and definitely by 48 hours—an athlete should begin nonweightbearing movement. For example, with ankle injuries movement from side to side (eversion, inversion) may be painful, but movement up and down (dorsal and plantar flexion) is not. So the latter type of movement can begin immediately.

With knee injuries, the quadriceps muscle becomes smaller because the knee joint is not moving. An athlete can do exercises to tighten the quadriceps without moving the knee joint. These should be done up to 100 times a day as soon as possible after injury.

7

Cardiovascular Conditioning

It takes 3 to 4 weeks for an athlete to get in shape and only 10 to 12 days to get out of shape. Many athletes are injured while recovering from an earlier injury because of lost conditioning.

Do everything you can to keep injured athletes in shape. Swimming is good for ankle and knee injuries because the body is lighter in water and does not bear weight. In the case of lower extremity injuries, stationary bikes and repetitive use of hand weights are good ways to maintain cardiovascular conditioning.

Jogging or running are permissible with upper extremity injuries as long as the activity does not cause pain.

Athletic Taping and Strapping

Athlete taping is a temporary measure, to be used for short periods only (i.e., practices and games). There are many ways to do taping. Each trainer has his or her own style, but there are some basic guidelines that apply to taping in general:

Uses of taping:
- Restrict motion of a joint, muscle, or tendon.
- Compress soft tissue.
- Hold bandages in place.
- Closure of lacerations.

Preparation for taping:
- Athlete should be in a comfortable position.
- You should be in a comfortable position.
- Body part to be wrapped should be adequately exposed.
- Remove body hair around injured area.
- Spray an adherent and follow with underwrap.

Application of tape:
- Follow the contour of the body in applying.
- Tape should be laid on, not pulled onto the skin.
- Tape should never tightly encircle soft tissue.
- Avoid wrinkles and folds that cause blisters.
- Avoid strapping tightly over bony prominences.

Removal of tape:
- Chemical removers can be used but are expensive.
- Tape cutters and bandage scissors are faster and cheaper.

- Applying Vaseline to bottom and tip of cutter or scissors allows them to slide under the tape.
- Start cutting on the side of the body opposite to the injured area; never cut over the injury.
- Keep cutting instrument perpendicular to the body.
- Remove adhesive by pulling tape slowly with one hand and pushing skin away with the other hand.
- Remove all residue and adherent from skin.
- Clean the body part and apply lotion containing lanolin.

More information about techniques for taping specific body parts can be obtained from the handbook *Athletic Uses of Adhesive Tape*, produced by the Johnson and Johnson Company. It has excellent photographs of tape being applied to thirteen different areas of the body as well as good general advice about taping.

Heat and Cold as Treatment

As a general rule, cold is preferable to heat for immediate use with acute injuries. In the case of chronic injuries and during the period following acute injuries, both heat and cold in combination are helpful. Heat and cold are **similar** in that both help decrease pain and spasm, but they **differ** in their effect on swelling and stretching. Knowing the important attributes of heat and cold can help you determine their appropriate use.

Heat increases stretchability. Muscles, tendons, and ligaments relax with heat, allowing them to stretch more during exercise. Heat reduces pain and decreases muscle spasm and stiffness. It increases cell metabolism, which increases blood flow. **When heat is applied to acute injuries, swelling increases because more blood comes to the site of the injury. Increased swelling is undesirable**.

Cold is an excellent pain reliever, because it reduces feeling in an area by decreasing the nerves' ability to conduct impulses. Cold lowers metabolism and blood flow, and therefore swelling decreases. Cooling also reduces spasms by inhibiting the muscles' ability to contract. But cold also increases stiffness and the inability to stretch.

When and How to Use Heat

Heat has limited use in sports medicine. Some trainers and physical therapists believe it should never be used. It certainly should never be used for acute injuries but may be of help in chronic injuries. Examples would be chronic back pain and overuse injuries that produce tightness in large muscles (quadriceps). In such cases, heat would help reduce the spasm and stiffness.

Heat can be applied by using hot water bottles, electric heating pads, or heat lamps. Make sure that the skin is protected and that heat is utilized for only a short period of time (10 to 15 minutes maximum).

When and How to Use Cold

Cold therapy is used for all acute injuries, such as contusions, strains, sprains, and broken bones. Cold stops bleeding and reduces pain, spasms, and swelling. Cold is also helpful for overuse syndromes, chronic pain, and in the repair stage of an injury.

Apply cold immediately with acute injuries and after exercise for chronic injuries. **Cold should be applied no longer than 20 minutes every 2 to 4 hours**. Skin being treated with cold passes through four stages—cold, burning, aching, and numbness. When it becomes numb, remove the ice. This usually takes 15 to 20 minutes.

Cold can be applied through the use of instant cold packs, ice bags, or ice cups. Cold packs get as cold as ice in three seconds, can be molded to the body, and are reusable. They are, however, more expensive than ice. Ice cubes can be placed in plastic bags or ice wraps and placed on an injured area for a minimum of 5 minutes and a maximum of 20 minutes.

Ice cups are made by freezing water in a paper cup. The top of the cup is peeled away, while the bottom protects the user's fingers. The ice is massaged into an injured area. Do not hold the ice directly over one spot for more than 30 seconds. Ice cups are ideal for post-exercise and chronic pain use.

Edward J. Shahady

4

Principles of Rehabilitation

Rehabilitation is one of the most overlooked parts of injury treatment. Many injuries recur during the recovery phase. Rehabilitation restores an injured or weakened area to its normal healthy state through exercise, which improves the strength, endurance, and flexibility of the muscles surrounding the injured area. Without rehabilitation the muscles remain weak, lengthening the recovery time and increasing the likelihood of reinjury. Rehabilitation is a necessary part of treating all injuries, regardless of severity.

Muscle grows and develops in response to stresses and forces placed upon it. **A change in these stresses or forces, such as occurs with decreased activity, causes a muscle to shorten and weaken**. Therapeutic exercises place stresses and forces on the muscle in order to prevent and/or overcome the loss of strength, endurance, and flexibility that occurs with injury.

Muscle Strength

Strength is the muscle or muscle group's ability to produce tension in relation to the demands placed upon it. Weak muscle has **atrophied** or decreased in size. With exercise, muscle **hypertrophies** or enlarges. The number of muscle fibers may actually increase in response to exercise. Strength increases because of a phenomenon known as recruitment, in which increased numbers of the units that make muscles contract are brought into use during the early phases of exercise, before muscles can hypertrophy.

Endurance

Endurance is the quality necessary for performing repeated tasks over a period of time. Muscular endurance is the ability to contract repeatedly or to generate tension and sustain that tension over a prolonged period of time. General body endurance or conditioning refers to the body's ability to maintain low-intensity exercise over an extended period. **Muscles and bodies that are not in shape are not strong and are therefore at greater risk of injury**.

Flexibility

In addition to strength and endurance, mobility or flexibility is necessary for an athlete to achieve maximum performance. Tightness occurs when a body part's normal motion is restricted in any way. **Trauma causes pain and inflammation, which lead to tightness or stiffness. This tightness causes more pain and inflammation**. Continuing to move injured joints and muscles is a preventative as well as a curative action. A classic example is the ankle sprain, in which restricted dorsiflexion (movement of the toes toward the shin) delays the recovery process.

Flexibility exercises must be specifically designed for a given body part. All exercises should start out at a lower weight and gradually increase the amount of resistance. These exercises should begin as soon as possible after an injury occurs, but they should not cause pain. Range-of-motion exercises should be started on the day of the injury to decrease stiffness. Resistance exercises are usually possible within two to three days after injury. Initial rehabilitation exercises are done 20 to 30 times, 2 to 3 times daily. As resistance is increased, the number of repetitions decreases and the exercises can be done once or twice a day.

Do not have the athlete perform exercises that cause pain and swelling. If these occur, decrease the weight being used by 25 to 50 percent to see if this helps. An injury is fully rehabilitated when there is normal motion, no swelling, and normal strength and when all physical activity can be performed without pain or restricted movement.

Each injury chapter in this guidebook contains exercises designed to condition muscles and prevent reinjury or to aid in the rehabilitation process. The chapter on flexibility should also be helpful for planning rehabilitation programs.

Edward J. Shahady

5

Flexibility

Flexibility is an important component of muscle fitness that unfortunately does not receive the emphasis it should as part of the athletic "routine." Flexibility exercises can do as much for strength and performance as weight training can. They also help prevent injuries, especially early in the season.

Flexibility refers to a joint's or group of joints' mobility or range of motion. A joint's ability to move depends on the muscles and ligaments that support it. Tight muscles reduce the range of motion, which in turn decreases the joint's ability to perform and increases the risk of injury.

Different sports use different muscle groups and so require different types of flexibility. For example, throwing sports require greater arm and shoulder flexibility. Football and basketball players, wrestlers, and weightlifters tend to have comparatively less flexibility, while gymnasts and swimmers have the most. Each sport develops specific muscle groups that are more flexible than other muscle groups. Swimmers, for instance, tend to have excellent ankle, shoulder, and trunk flexibility.

Types of Stretching

The development of flexibility is contingent on overload, which means that a muscle must be stretched beyond its normal length in order to increase flexibility. **There are four types of stretching: passive, passive with an assist, active, and proprioceptive neuromuscular facilitation (PNF)**. Passive stretching is preferred for flexibility training, but the other types also have their places.

Passive stretching is also known as static or slow stretching. It is a slow, sustained stretch that places the muscle in a lengthened position and holds it there for a few seconds. This method does not produce muscle soreness and is less likely to provoke injury from overstretching.

Passive stretching with an assist: Sometimes passive stretching alone will not achieve the desired increase in muscle flexibility. In such cases, an assist can increase the force on the muscle. For example, standing and reaching for your toes, as opposed to sitting and reaching for them, allows gravity to provide an assist. A partner can also assist by pushing forward against your shoulders as you try to touch your toes from a sitting position.

Active stretching, also known as dynamic, fast, or bouncing stretching, involves bouncing or jerking to gain the momentum needed to produce overstretching. A second person can assist. **Injury and muscle soreness are more likely with active stretching**, so this method should only be used by experienced athletes who have good flexibility.

Proprioceptive neuromuscular facilitation (PNF) is an assisted passive stretching procedure in which the muscle is contracted before it is stretched. Then a passive assisted stretch is applied while the antagonist muscle (muscle going against the function of the other) is contracted. Although this method is believed to enhance the effects of passive stretching, there is no proof that it is better than passive stretching alone.

Stretching Exercises

Do not do all your stretching exercises at one time; instead, spread them out over the course of the day. Stretching should be done every day, sometimes three to six times a day. The length of time taken for a stretch should be at least 5 seconds. More time could lead to pain. Stretch until you begin to feel a pull in your muscle. Three sets of 6 to 25 repetitions each are recommended. The following stretching exercises can be utilized:

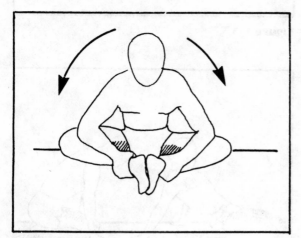

Figure 5-1

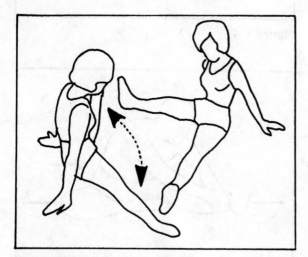

Figure 5-2

Groin Stretch

• Sit with your feet together and heels pulled toward your body. Grasp each ankle and press your knees downward with your elbows (Fig. 5-1). Figure 5-2 notes an alternate way to stretch the groin muscles. Sit facing a partner with legs spread apart and feet touching. Aid each other in gradual stretching by pushing legs further apart. The width of the stretch should increase each time. Hold the stretch for 8 seconds and repeat 3 times.

Gastroc–Lower-Back Stretch

• Sit on the floor, legs in front of you with knees bent, and grasp the soles of your feet. Gradually straighten your legs while keeping your head close to your knees (Fig. 5-3). Hold for 20 seconds and repeat 3 times.

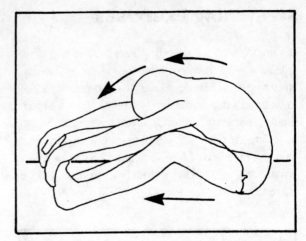

Figure 5-3

Ankle and Quad Stretch

• Kneel with your toes pointed behind you. First place your hands on the floor in front of you and then lean back with your hands behind you (Fig. 5-4). Do slowly and with control. Hold while leaning backward for 20 seconds and repeat 3 times.

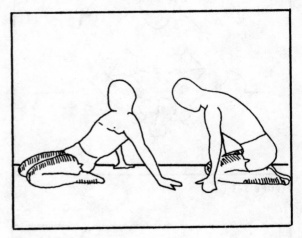

Figure 5-4

Hamstring and Lower-Back Stretch

• Sit with one leg straight in front of you and place the sole of the other foot against the inside of your thigh (Fig. 5-5). Bend forward, keeping the leg straight, and hold for 20 seconds. Repeat 3 times for each leg.

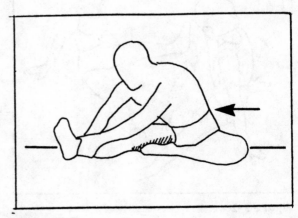

Figure 5-5

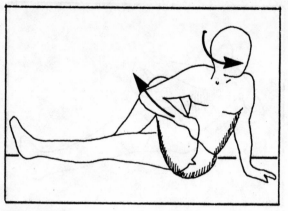

Figure 5-6

Trunk Twister

• Sit with one leg straight and the other leg crossed over at the knee (Fig. 5-6). Place one hand behind you and the other arm up against the crossed leg. Turn your neck toward the hand behind you and push on the crossed leg with your other elbow. Hold for 20 seconds and repeat 3 times for each leg.

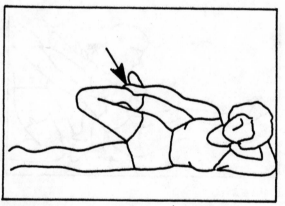

Figure 5-7

Quadriceps, Hip, and Ankle Stretch

• While lying on one side, support your head with the lower hand and bend your upper leg. Grab the top of the foot of the bent leg and pull it toward your buttock as shown (Fig. 5-7). Hold for 20 seconds and repeat 3 times with each leg.

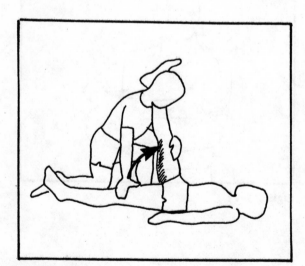

Figure 5-8

Hamstring Stretch

• While lying on your back, have a partner keep one of your legs straight and the other leg extended upward against his or her shoulder (Fig. 5-8). Begin the exercise by pushing your leg downward against your partner's shoulder. Hold your contraction for 3 to 5 seconds. Your partner should then push upward against your leg for 15 seconds. Repeat 3 times.

Upper Hamstring Hip Stretch

• Lie down and, with one hand on your knee and the other on the outside of your ankle, pull your leg toward your chest (Fig. 5-9). Pull until you feel a strain in the back of the upper leg. Hold for 20 seconds, then repeat 3 times with each leg.

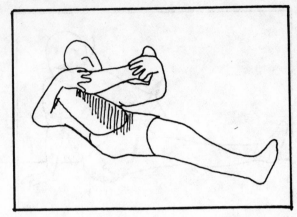

Figure 5-9

Shoulder Stretches

• Sit with your arms extended to each side. Have a partner sit behind you and pull your arms backward while you pull forward (Fig. 5-10). Hold for 8 seconds and repeat 3 times.

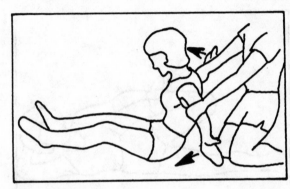

Figure 5-10

• With one hand, grasp your other arm just above the elbow and pull the shoulder down and then across the chest (Fig. 5-11). Hold for 25 seconds and repeat 3 times for each arm.

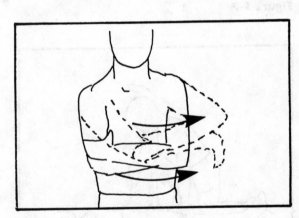

Figure 5-11

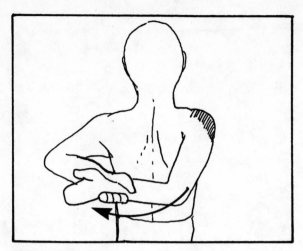

Figure 5-12

• Place one arm behind your back and pull it slowly across your back with the other hand (Fig. 5-12). Hold for 25 seconds and repeat 3 times for both arms.

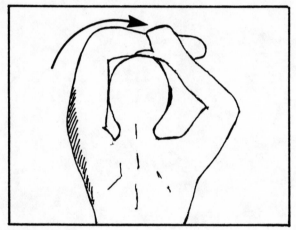

Figure 5-13

• Place arm above your head and grasp the wrist with your other hand. Pull the arm across and behind your head (Fig. 5-13). Hold for 25 seconds and repeat 3 times for both arms.

NOTE: From the very first, establish good habits by stressing proper stretching techniques. Stretching should be an important part of practices early in the season, as players are not in top condition. Their muscles are liable to be tight, making them more susceptible to injury.

Timothy J. Ives

Medications for Sports Injuries

Aspirin, acetaminophen, and ibuprofen are the three types of medications commonly used for the pain and inflammation associated with sports injuries. All three of these drugs provide pain relief, and aspirin and ibuprofen help reduce inflammation in such injuries as tendinitis, bursitis, and overuse syndromes. All can be obtained without a prescription, making them readily accessible for use by athletes, and all can be recommended by coaches, trainers, and physicians. **Though these medications are relatively safe, it is wise to know how to use them most effectively and to be aware of some of the side effects that can occur**.

Acetaminophen, commonly marketed as Tylenol, is excellent for the pain of acute injuries and can be combined with aspirin and ibuprofen. Two adult-strength tablets (325 mg each) or one double-strength tablet (500 mg) every four hours is an appropriate dose for pain relief. Other than an occasional upset stomach, the side effects from acetaminophen are minimal to nonexistent. Adult dosages can be given to anyone over twelve years of age or weighing more than 120 pounds.

Aspirin is an excellent drug for both pain and inflammation and is inexpensive compared to ibuprofen. The usual adult dose is two 325 mg aspirins four to six times a day. Aspirin can cause an upset stomach and also diarrhea, dizziness, and headache. Some of these side effects can be lessened if the aspirin is taken with meals or is enteric-coated (e.g., Ecotrin and similar products). Allergic reactions to aspirin may sometimes cause asthma or hives. Aside from the upset stomach, however, these side effects are uncommon. **Most athletes do not get relief from aspirin because they take less than the necessary dosage**.

Ibuprofen comes in several forms—Advil, Nuprin, Motrin, and Medipren are the most widely known. Ibuprofen is a nonsteroidal anti-inflammatory drug (NSAID) and costs more than aspirin. The dosage for ibuprofen can be as much as sixteen 200 mg tablets a day; however, this high dosage is usually reserved for a 250-pound lineman. **Two 200 mg tablets 4 times a day is an average dose**. The effect of the drug decreases in three to four hours, so it is important to take it frequently. The side effects are similar to those of aspirin, but stomach distress is much less common with ibuprofen. Dizziness, headache, and diarrhea can occur in 3 to 5 percent of those taking it. A person who is allergic to aspirin may also be allergic to ibuprofen. An asthmatic patient should be warned that ibuprofen can cause an increase in asthmatic symptoms.

Points to Remember

1. **Low doses of aspirin and ibuprofen (one or two tablets) provide pain relief but do not reduce inflammation very effectively. Higher doses (ten aspirin a day, eight ibuprofen a day) reduce inflammation**.

2. Acute soft-tissue injuries in which swelling is sec-

ondary to bleeding are not a contraindication to the use of ibuprofen or other nonsteroidal anti-inflammatory drugs. In fact, these drugs have been shown actually to reduce the healing time and hasten the athlete's return to activity.

3. Aspirin and ibuprofen should not be used before or during exercise in order to prevent or decrease eventual pain.

4. Renal damage is not a problem for a well-hydrated athlete, but aspirin and ibuprofen should not be used if the athlete is dehydrated.

5. Discuss medication use with your team physician. Knowing how to use the drugs will greatly boost your effectiveness.

Section 2

Diagnosis and Treatment of Specific Injuries

Guide to Rapid Diagnosis

Knowing the location of the pain and how the injury occurred can help you make a rapid diagnosis. The following tables take this information into account and direct you to the proper page.

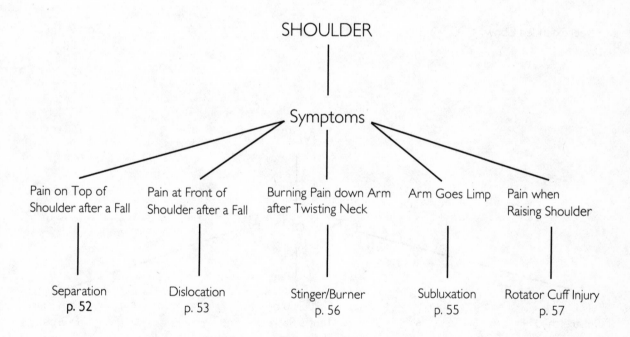

SHOULDER

Symptoms

Pain on Top of Shoulder after a Fall	Pain at Front of Shoulder after a Fall	Burning Pain down Arm after Twisting Neck	Arm Goes Limp	Pain when Raising Shoulder
Separation p. 52	Dislocation p. 53	Stinger/Burner p. 56	Subluxation p. 55	Rotator Cuff Injury p. 57

ELBOW

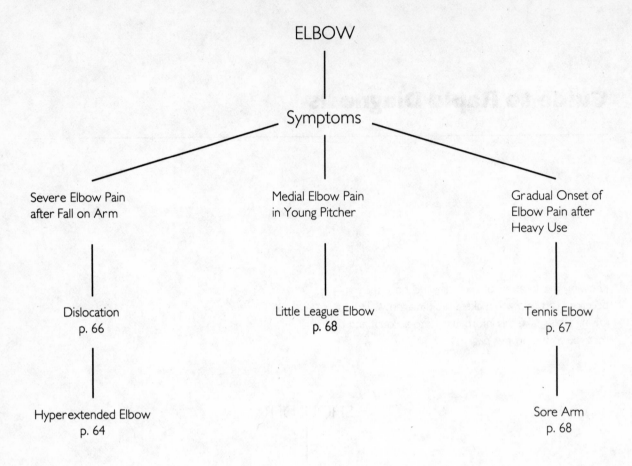

Symptoms

Severe Elbow Pain
after Fall on Arm

Medial Elbow Pain
in Young Pitcher

Gradual Onset of
Elbow Pain after
Heavy Use

Dislocation
p. 66

Little League Elbow
p. 68

Tennis Elbow
p. 67

Hyperextended Elbow
p. 64

Sore Arm
p. 68

WRIST

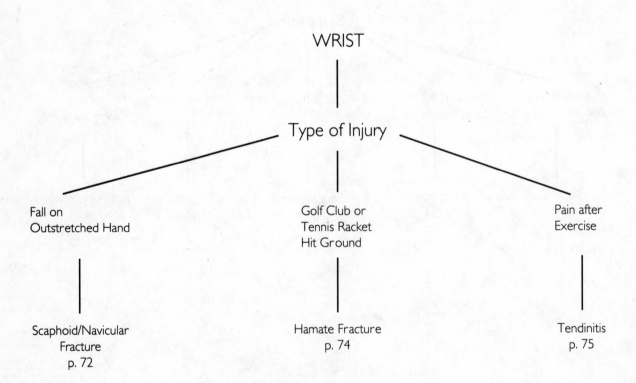

Type of Injury

Fall on
Outstretched Hand

Golf Club or
Tennis Racket
Hit Ground

Pain after
Exercise

Scaphoid/Navicular
Fracture
p. 72

Hamate Fracture
p. 74

Tendinitis
p. 75

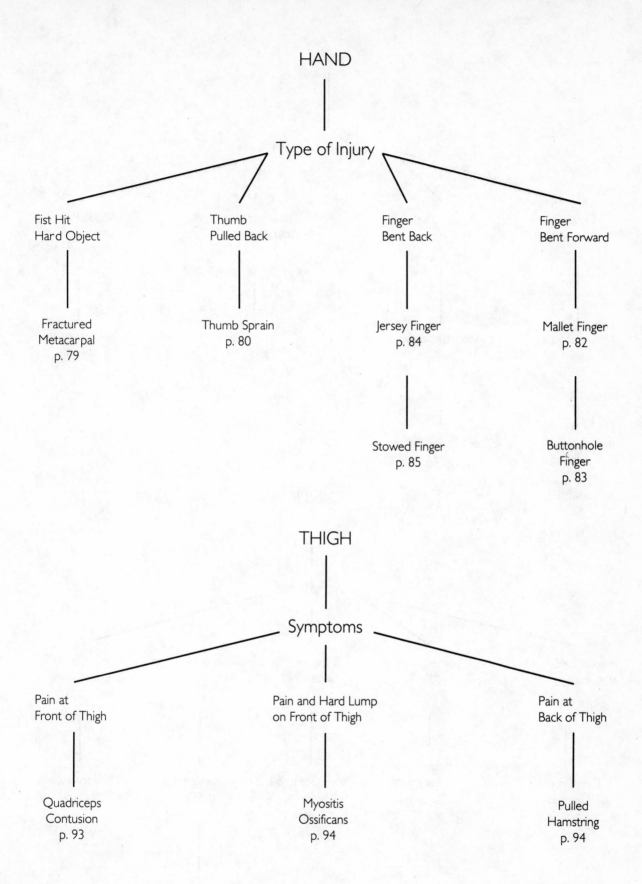

HAND

Type of Injury

Fist Hit
Hard Object

Fractured
Metacarpal
p. 79

Thumb
Pulled Back

Thumb Sprain
p. 80

Finger
Bent Back

Jersey Finger
p. 84

Stowed Finger
p. 85

Finger
Bent Forward

Mallet Finger
p. 82

Buttonhole
Finger
p. 83

THIGH

Symptoms

Pain at
Front of Thigh

Quadriceps
Contusion
p. 93

Pain and Hard Lump
on Front of Thigh

Myositis
Ossificans
p. 94

Pain at
Back of Thigh

Pulled
Hamstring
p. 94

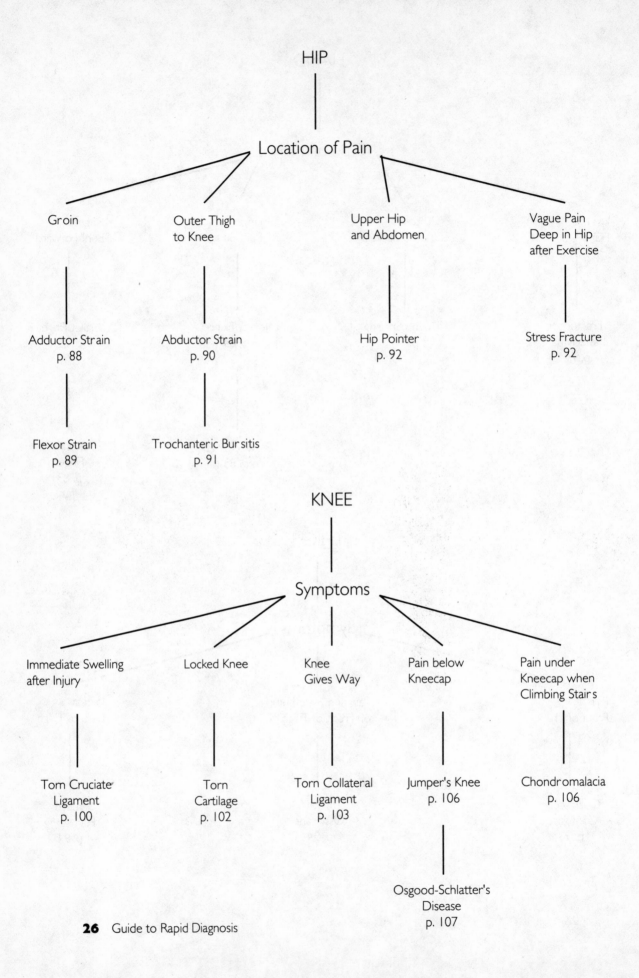

HIP

Location of Pain

Groin

Outer Thigh
to Knee

Upper Hip
and Abdomen

Vague Pain
Deep in Hip
after Exercise

Adductor Strain
p. 88

Abductor Strain
p. 90

Hip Pointer
p. 92

Stress Fracture
p. 92

Flexor Strain
p. 89

Trochanteric Bursitis
p. 91

KNEE

Symptoms

Immediate Swelling
after Injury

Locked Knee

Knee
Gives Way

Pain below
Kneecap

Pain under
Kneecap when
Climbing Stairs

Torn Cruciate
Ligament
p. 100

Torn
Cartilage
p. 102

Torn Collateral
Ligament
p. 103

Jumper's Knee
p. 106

Chondromalacia
p. 106

Osgood-Schlatter's
Disease
p. 107

LOWER EXTREMITY

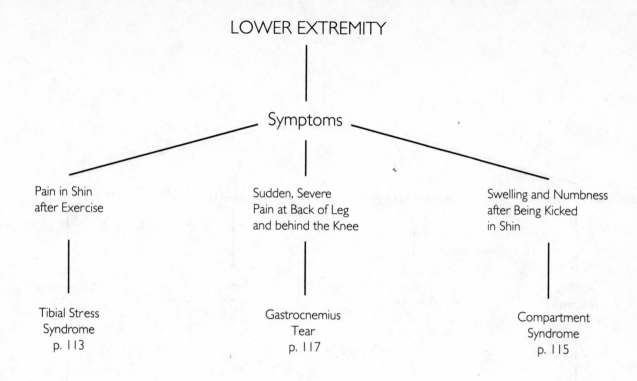

Symptoms

Pain in Shin
after Exercise

Sudden, Severe
Pain at Back of Leg
and behind the Knee

Swelling and Numbness
after Being Kicked
in Shin

Tibial Stress
Syndrome
p. 113

Gastrocnemius
Tear
p. 117

Compartment
Syndrome
p. 115

ANKLE

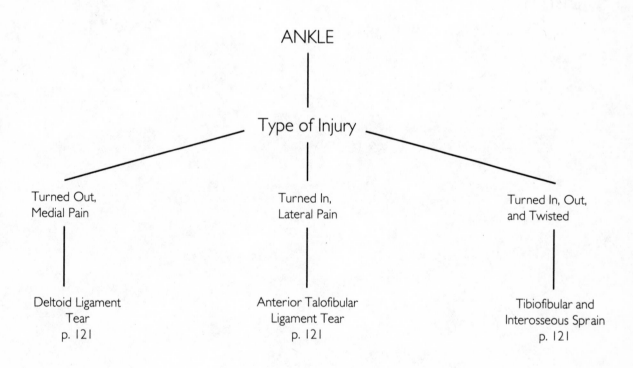

Type of Injury

Turned Out,
Medial Pain

Turned In,
Lateral Pain

Turned In, Out,
and Twisted

Deltoid Ligament
Tear
p. 121

Anterior Talofibular
Ligament Tear
p. 121

Tibiofibular and
Interosseous Sprain
p. 121

FOOT

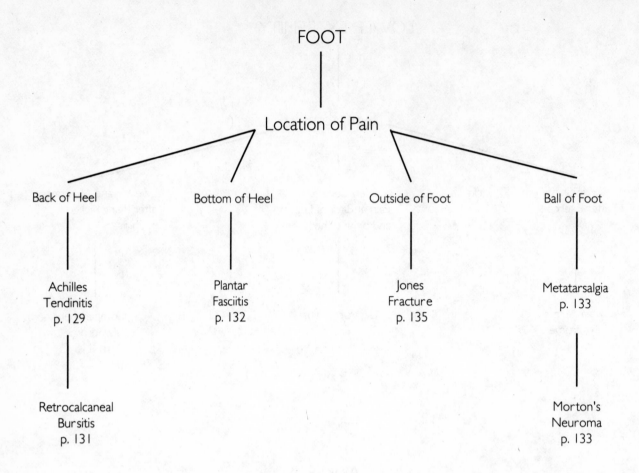

Location of Pain

Back of Heel

Bottom of Heel

Outside of Foot

Ball of Foot

Achilles
Tendinitis
p. 129

Plantar
Fasciitis
p. 132

Jones
Fracture
p. 135

Metatarsalgia
p. 133

Retrocalcaneal
Bursitis
p. 131

Morton's
Neuroma
p. 133

Edward J. Shahady

Head and
Neck Injuries

Injuries to the head and neck can be extremely painful and frightening to an athlete, and they are also the most alarming and difficult of injuries to evaluate. These injuries range from superficial cuts and bruises to life-threatening fractures. A severe head or neck injury can leave an athlete unconscious and/or temporarily paralyzed. Damage to the brain or spinal cord can cause permanent paralysis or possibly death. Because the functions of the head and neck are so vital and yet so vulnerable, adults involved in high school athletics—and particularly in such high risk sports as football—must have a thorough understanding of head and neck injuries: how to prevent them, how to recognize them, and what to do when one occurs. Neck injuries are often more severe and should be diagnosed first when combined with a head injury. Any head injury exam should include an evaluation of the neck. With head and neck injuries, ignorance can be extremely harmful and even fatal.

Contact sports such as football account for the vast majority of head and neck injuries in high school athletics. The 1976 rules change making butt blocking, face tackling, and spearing illegal has done a great deal to reduce the occurrence of head and neck injuries in football. Football coaches should constantly stress to their athletes the importance of keeping their heads up when blocking or tackling. **The head should never be the initial point of contact**.

Head Injuries

Cuts, **bumps**, and **concussions** are the most common injuries to the head and may occur simultaneously. Whenever an athlete receives a blow to the head sufficient to break the skin or create a bump, be sure to check for signs of a concussion as well.

Cuts

Because the head has a very rich blood supply, even small cuts tend to bleed heavily. You should take the following steps with head cuts:
• Try to stop the bleeding initially by applying pressure to the cut with a sterile gauze pad. Most bleeding stops within three to four minutes. A lot of blood often frightens a young athlete. Keep calm and reassure the athlete that the cut is not serious.
• Once the bleeding from a small cut stops, clean the cut with soap and water and allow the athlete to resume activity. Watch the cut closely for signs of infection, which include increased redness and tenderness around the cut and a yellowish liquid leaking from the cut. Refer an athlete with an infection to a physician.
• A large cut with more severe bleeding may require stitches. After the athlete has seen a physician, check the cut or stitches periodically for signs of infection. **Do**

not attempt to remove the stitches without prior instruction from the team physician.

Bumps

Bumps, or goose eggs, occur fairly frequently. If there are no signs of concussion, very little need be done. Place ice packs over the bump for 15 to 20 minutes. If the athlete loses consciousness or exhibits unusual behavior following the injury, follow the guidelines listed under "Concussions."

Concussions

Description

Concussions result from a blow to the head that causes an athlete to become dazed or, in severe cases, to lose consciousness. Concussions are graded from one (1) to five (5), according to severity. The first three grades are very common. The exam is the same for all five grades.

Complete Concussion Exam

• Check for a pulse and make sure the athlete is breathing. If the athlete is unconscious but has a pulse and no apparent problems breathing, there is no need to hurry. The athlete will begin to recover in a short time.
• **Do not allow the athlete to move before you examine the neck for a fracture**.
• Check the athlete's arms and legs to be sure they have equal strength and feeling.
• Be sure the athlete is aware of the date, time, and place and the names of people in the vicinity.
• Check for **retrograde amnesia**—the inability to remember things that happened before the injury (e.g., score in the game or identity of the opposing team).
• Also check for **post-event amnesia**—the inability to remember what happened right after the injury (e.g., being dazed, who was talking to him, or who walked her off the field).

Grade 1

Symptoms

• The athlete does not lose consciousness but is dazed or confused for 5 to 15 minutes.

• Athletes often describe this sensation as "having their bell rung" or "getting dinged."
• The athlete may experience mild unsteadiness in walking but displays no other symptoms such as amnesia.

Treatment

• Have the athlete rest until his or her head clears.
• Allow the athlete to return to full activity upon regaining complete lucidity.
• Watch for recurring symptoms.

Grade 2

Symptoms

• Similar to Grade 1, except that the athlete **experiences memory loss**. Upon regaining lucidity the athlete experiences post-event amnesia (see above).

Treatment

• This athlete should not return to activity the same day.
• Watch the athlete closely for 3 to 4 days. Most athletes have no trouble, but one who acts unusual or who begins to develop bouts of forgetfulness, tiredness, or headaches should be evaluated by a physician.
• **Postconcussion syndrome**, or "athlete's migraine," often occurs after Grade 2 concussions. With this, athletes experience recurrent headaches, an inability to concentrate, and irritability, and such athletes need to see a physician before returning to activity.

Grade 3

Symptoms

• Similar to Grades 1 and 2, with the addition of retrograde amnesia (see above).
• Athlete does not lose consciousness.

Treatment

• Athletes who display symptoms of a Grade 3 concussion should not return to activity and should be evaluated by a physician.
• Observe these athletes for postconcussion syndrome and unusual behavior for 1 to 2 weeks. If they are doing well, the physician will usually allow them to return to play after 4 to 7 days.

Grade 4

Symptoms

• The athlete is "knocked out" or unconscious but usually recovers within seconds or minutes.

• The athlete emerges from the coma confused and disoriented for a few moments, then becomes fully alert but cannot remember the injury or confusion and also has retrograde amnesia.

Treatment

• Because these athletes are unsteady for a time, they should be carried off the field on a stretcher or spine board. If one insists on walking, have him or her slowly rise from lying flat to a sitting and then a standing position. If there is any sign of unsteadiness, insist on using a stretcher.

• Any athlete who loses consciousness must see a physician **as soon as possible**.

• Do not allow an athlete who has exhibited these symptoms to return to play even if the player seems fully recovered. Such an athlete may have bleeding in the brain and could feel well for 20 to 30 minutes before collapsing again.

Grade 5

Symptoms

• The athlete is unconscious and does not regain full consciousness. A concussion this severe rarely occurs but, because of its severity, coaches and trainers need to be fully prepared for it.

• The athlete remains disoriented upon regaining consciousness.

Treatment

• Place the athlete on a spine board or stretcher. **Protect the cervical spine as if it were broken. Make sure the athlete is strapped securely to the spine board**.

• Get the athlete to the nearest emergency room. If an ambulance with trained personnel is not available, you should accompany the athlete to the hospital. The bed of a pickup truck or a van are alternate means of transportation.

Neck Injuries

Most neck injuries consist of minor strains to the muscles and ligaments. Any neck injury, however, is potentially very serious. When examining an athlete who has sustained a neck injury, you should always check for serious injuries as well as minor ones. A complete neck exam includes **palpation** (touching) of the vertebrae and muscles, **active and passive neck movement**, evaluation of the **ability to feel** in the arms and hand, and tests for **arm strength**.

There are seven bones in the neck, which are called **cervical vertebrae** (Fig. 7-1). The major muscles attached to the neck are the **sternoclidomastoid** and **trapezius** (Fig. 7-2). The cervical vertebrae protect the spinal cord and the cervical nerves. Damage to the cervical vertebrae can hurt the spinal cord and cervical nerves as well. However, broken bones in the neck do not always produce injuries to the nerves and spinal cord.

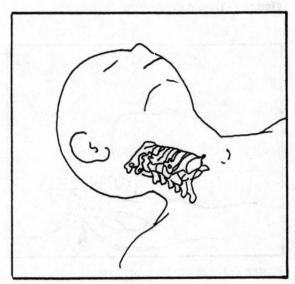

Figure 7-1. Cervical vertebrae

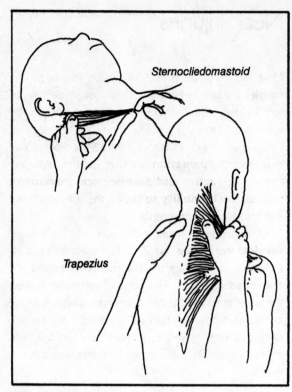

Figure 7-2. Muscles of the neck

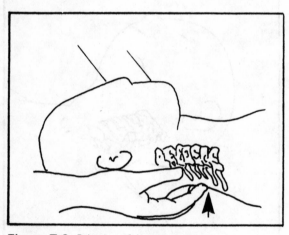

Figure 7-3. Palpation of the vertebrae

Complete Neck Exam

• Palpate (touch) the vertebrae and muscles (Fig. 7-3). Determine the location of pain. Pain over the cervical spine indicates a possible fracture. When the symptoms indicate a possible fracture or nerve damage, follow the procedure outlined in the section below entitled "Broken Bones in the Neck." Pain over the muscles indicates a sprain, tear, or contusion. Check also for a hematoma (collection of blood), which feels like a hardening lump.

• Assess the nerves of the cervical spine. Weakness or loss of feeling in the shoulders and arms can indicate possible nerve damage. If the athlete complains of weakness in or the inability to move arms and legs in addition to neck pain, **do not have the athlete perform any neck movements**.

• Tests for **strength**:

Shoulder muscles—use the deltoid and the rotator cuff strength tests (see Chapter 11, "Shoulder Injuries").

Upper arm—Biceps and triceps and brachioradialis strength testing (Figs. 7-4, 7-5).

Forearm—Wrist extension and wrist flexion (Figs. 7-6, 7-7).

• Tests for **sensation** (feeling):

Do not use anything that could break the skin and lead to infection. Use an open paper clip. Have the athlete look away from the points being touched and tell if one or both of the points are felt. This is known as "two point discrimination." Test the tips of all fingers and the thumb as well as both sides of the upper and lower arm (Fig. 7-8). It is a good idea to practice this ahead of time.

• If palpation reveals no pain, ask the athlete to nod the head, touch chin to chest, chin to left and right shoulder, and left ear to left shoulder and right ear to right shoulder (**active neck movements**). If the athlete can perform these motions without pain, there is probably no fracture. If the athlete is unable to do any one of these motions because of pain, treat as if a bone is broken.

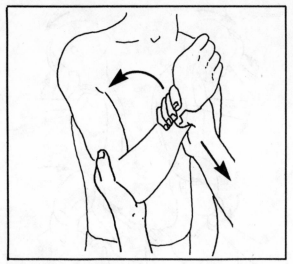

Figure 7-4. Strength test for biceps and brachioradialis

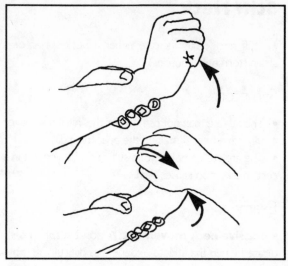

Figure 7-6. Test for wrist extension

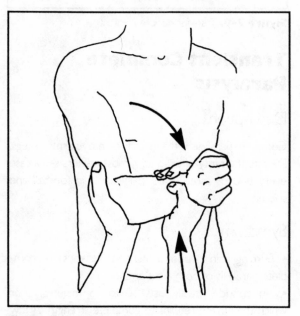

Figure 7-5. Strength test for triceps

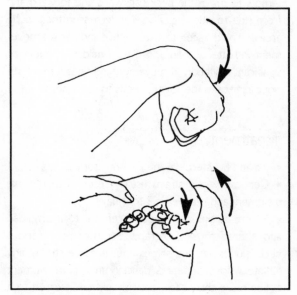

Figure 7-7. Test for wrist flexion

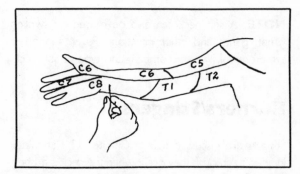

Figure 7-8. Test for sensation (feeling)

Stiff Neck

A "stiff neck" may indicate either a neck sprain or a strain (torn neck muscles).

Symptoms

• The athlete may not remember the initial trauma, or it may have been sustained the preceding day.
• The athlete complains of a stiff neck. Movement in a certain direction causes pain.

Exam

• **Passive neck movement**. A possible sprain is indicated when the athlete experiences difficulty in moving the neck in one or more directions.
• **Active neck movement**. Resist the athlete's attempts to move the neck backward and forward and from side to side (Fig. 7-9). Tenderness in the muscle area and mild discomfort with active and passive movement indicate a strain. More than mild discomfort or significant limitation of movement indicates a more serious injury and the athlete needs to see a physician.

Treatment

• Ice and nonsteroidal anti-inflammatories.
• Cervical muscle strains usually respond to minimal treatment and recover in 3 to 4 days.
• Severe strains may require referral to a physician and intense physical therapy. Because more serious neck injuries can sometimes appear to be strains, any athlete who experiences difficulty in neck movement lasting more than a few days should be referred to a physician.

NOTE: A stiff neck can also be caused by swollen lymph glands and other infections. Fever and other symptoms of illness accompany this type of stiff neck.

Burners/Stingers

Stingers are discussed fully in Chapter 11 ("Shoulder Injuries"). Although they occur when the neck is pushed to one side, stretching the neck nerves, the symptoms include shoulder pain and weakness and a burning sensation shooting through the arm.

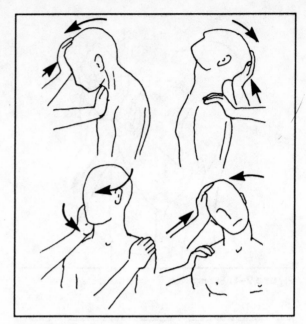

Figure 7-9. Tests for neck movement

Transient Complete Paralysis

Description

Complete paralysis is the inability to move arms or legs. Despite the rarity of this injury, most trainers see a case every two or three years, particularly in football and soccer.

Symptoms

• Burning pain in both arms, and weakness or complete paralysis of both arms and legs.
• An episode usually lasts 10 to 15 minutes, after which the athlete returns to complete strength. A few cases have lasted up to 36 hours.

Exam

• Palpate the neck and check neck movement to see if either produces pain.

Treatment

• Have the athlete checked by a physician. Transient loss of feeling and movement may be due to a narrowing of the column through which the spinal cord passes. It is important that athletes who suffer this injury receive physician evaluation before returning to participation in contact sports.

Broken Bones in the Neck

Description

Broken bones in the neck are not always associated with nerve damage, but when a bone breaks, the possibility of nerve damage exists. The first priority is to **protect the athlete from nerve damage**. The athlete may be unconscious, and you should proceed with treatment as if the neck is broken until it is proved otherwise. A conscious athlete is likely to be very frightened and will need reassurance. For the athlete's sake, learn ahead of time how to evaluate and treat possible neck fractures. Practice with the team doctor and student trainers so that all know and understand their roles. It is an excellent idea to have the routine written down so that it can be easily reviewed and passed along to others.

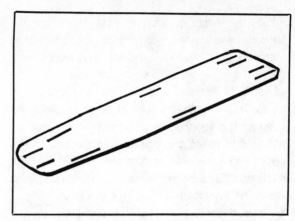
Figure 7-10. Spine board

Symptoms

• Moderate to severe pain in the neck immediately following violent contact such as a tackle or a fall to the floor that hyperextends or hyperflexes the neck.
• The athlete may be unconscious or lying very still.

Exam

• Do not move the athlete until the exam is completed.
• If the athlete is unconscious, check for pulse and breathing.
• Determine the location of the pain by touching the neck over the area of the cervical spine (see Fig. 7-3). Pain over the cervical spine indicates a possible fracture.

NOTE: A football player's helmet makes a neck examination difficult, **but do not remove the helmet, as it provides stabilization**.

Treatment

• Allow the athlete a few moments to recover from the initial scare. Make certain the injury is not a stinger or a sprain.
• Remember that your goal is to protect the spinal cord and nerve roots from injury or further injury.
• Place a spine board or fracture board (Fig. 7-10) next to the athlete.
• A medical team composed of four members can move an athlete who is face down by using a method called "log rolling" (Fig. 7-11). The medical team's leader

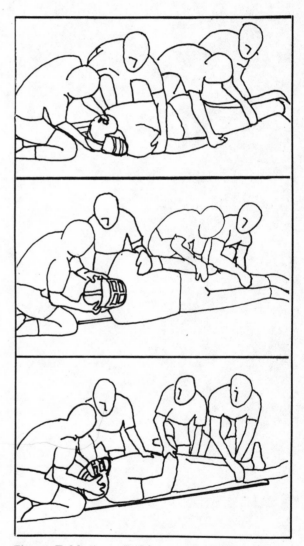
Figure 7-11. "Log rolling" for suspected broken neck

(ideally the trainer or team physician) maneuvers the athlete's head and gives commands. The other three members roll the athlete, and then the leader helps them lift and carry. Position one team member at the athlete's shoulders, one at the hips, and one at the knees. Tuck the athlete's arms at his or her sides and bring the legs together. Keep the body in a straight position while rolling the athlete onto the board. The leader keeps the head immobilized by applying slight traction and by using the crossed-arm technique, which allows the arms to unwind during the roll.

- If the athlete to be transported is lying face up, the medical team assumes the same stations, rolls the fully protected athlete onto one side, and slides the fracture board underneath. Helmets should be left on. Face masks can be removed by cutting the plastic loops. The athlete's head should be stabilized with a strap, if there is one attached to the spine board, or with several strips of adhesive tape. Ambulance drivers may also have sandbags or straps.

Prevention

Emphasize proper training and playing techniques.

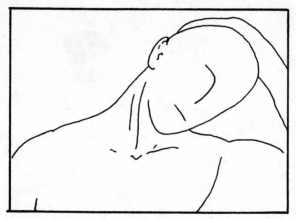
Figure 7-12. Neck strengthening

Neck Exercises

Neck Stretching

• Sit or stand with arms to your side. Move your neck slowly forward, backward, left, and right. Your ears should touch your shoulders during the left and right motions. Hold each movement to a count of five. Do this for 20 repetitions before starting neck-strengthening exercises.

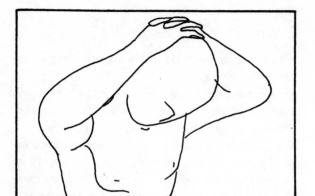
Figure 7-13. Neck strengthening

Neck Strengthening

• Sit or stand and push your head in different directions using your hands for resistance (Figs. 7-12, 7-13). Hold each repetition for 5 seconds. Do this exercise 10 times in each direction.

Teresa M. Shields

Eye Injuries

The National Society to Prevent Blindness estimates that about 167,000 eye injuries occur annually in school-aged children, with two-thirds of these being sports related. Sports-related accidents have accounted for 23 percent of all eye injury hospitalizations; 90 percent or more of these injuries could have been prevented by the use of proper protective eyewear and other safety precautions. Coaches, athletic directors, and team physicians should be familiar with current guidelines and equipment designed to prevent eye injuries and be prepared to properly evaluate athletic eye injuries.

Blow to the Eye

Description

Fingers or elbows and balls or other pieces of equipment all can injure the eye. Wrestling, basketball, volleyball, lacrosse, and soccer are some of the sports associated with direct blows to the eye.

Symptoms

• Immediate pain and a high degree of anxiety are almost always present.
• The athlete usually covers the eye with his or her hand.
• The athlete may complain of seeing spots or stars and of a decrease in vision.

Exam

• Have the athlete sit down. Do not begin your exam until he or she is relaxed.
• Test the vision in both eyes. Cover up one eye and have the athlete read any available print (e.g., game program or newspaper). Test each eye separately.
• Inspect the eye (Fig. 8-1). Look at the periorbital area (area around the eye), the sclera (white of the eye), the iris (the colored part of the eye), and the pupil (the dark circle in the middle of the eye) and inspect for any swelling, cuts, or a difference between the injured and the uninjured eye. A penlight or small flashlight can help with the inspection.
• Test for pupillary reflexes (Fig. 8-2). Have the athlete focus on a distant object and then shine a light into each pupil. The pupils on both sides should constrict (become smaller).
• Check eyeball movement. The eyeball moves in six directions (Fig. 8-3). Have the athlete follow your finger to see if the eye moves in all directions. Compare movement in the injured eye to that of the normal eye and ask if the athlete experiences double vision during any of these movements.
• Palpate (touch) the periorbital area. Severe pain may indicate a broken bone.

Treatment

• Your main goal in treating eye injuries is to be sure that nothing serious is wrong. If vision is normal, the pupils react to light, eye movements are normal, and your inspection and palpation of the eye reveal nothing abnormal, then you can assume that nothing serious

38

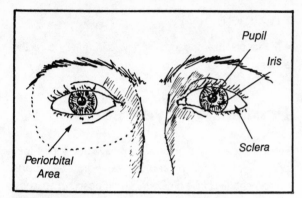

Figure 8-1. Front view of eyes

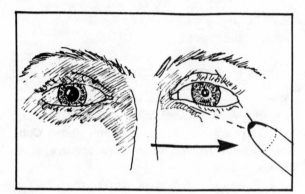

Figure 8-2. Pupil reacting to light

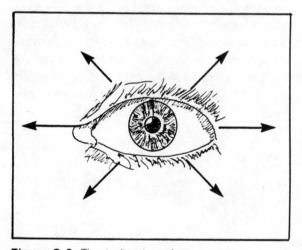

Figure 8-3. The six directions of eye movement

has occurred, but any deviation from normal warrants evaluation by a physician.

• Usually, an ice pack, reassurance, and time are all the treatment needed. If swelling is severe enough to obstruct vision, the athlete probably should not compete until the swelling has diminished.

Something in the Eye

Description

Dust or dirt may get caught in a player's eye, or the outer eye may be scratched, resulting in the sensation of having something in the eye. Outdoor sports and contact sports have the highest incidence of this type of injury.

Symptoms

• Eye pain
• Tearing
• Sensation of having something in the eye
• Frequent blinking of the eyelids

Exam

• Inspect the eye. If you see the piece of dirt, have the athlete blink and see if the object moves to the corner of the eye. A Q-tip can then be used to remove the dirt.
• Check under the lower lid. Ask the athlete to look up while you place traction on the lid margin.
• Check under the upper lid. Place a Q-tip at the base of the eyelid and grasp the eyelashes with your index finger and thumb. Roll the lid margin over the Q-tip by pulling up on the eyelashes and pushing down on the Q-tip (Fig. 8-4).

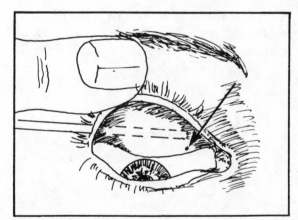

Figure 8-4. Exposing upper lid to check for foreign body

Treatment

• If the piece of dirt is visible under the upper or lower lids or in the corner of the eye, it can be removed with a Q-tip. Moistening the Q-tip with a sterile irrigating solution sometimes makes the removal easier.

• Pieces of dirt that are stuck in the middle of the eye and don't move when the eye is moved need to be taken out by a physician.

• After you have removed the piece of dirt, the sensation of something in the eye should be gone. If the sensation remains, the athlete may have scratched his or her cornea. A scratched cornea may also be the cause when an athlete complains of something in the eye but nothing can be found. Corneal scratches should be evaluated by a physician.

Pinkeye

Description

Pinkeye, also called **conjunctivitis**, is an infection or inflammation of the eyelids.

Symptoms

• A gritty or sandy feeling in the eyes and increased watering.

Exam

• Look for yellow discharge and bloodshot eyes.

• Check for eye pain or photophobia (light hurts the eyes). Either of these symptoms associated with pinkeye indicates a more serious problem.

Treatment

• Eyedrops prescribed by a physician usually cure the problem.

Protective Eyewear

Several international organizations have developed specific guidelines for protective eyewear. The Sports Equipment Certification Council (composed of coaches, scientists, physicians, athletes, and manufacturers) tests equipment and sets industry standards for all forms of protective sports equipment, including eyewear. The council affixes its seal to safety equipment, identifying products that meet the standards.

Contact Lenses and Eyeglasses

Athletes often prefer contact lenses because they allow normal peripheral vision, do not fog, and are considered more cosmetically appealing than glasses. **Contact lenses, however, offer no protection against injury**. Contact wearers should wear the standard protective eyewear recommended for their sport in addition to contacts.

Streetwear eyeglasses should not be worn for athletic activities. These lenses meet FDA specifications only for ordinary daily hazards. Industrial safety glasses meet higher impact-resistance specifications and are available in a variety of lens and frame styles. Polycarbonate lenses have the highest impact resistance currently available and can be obtained as either prescription or nonprescription lenses.

Chest, Thorax, and Abdomen Injuries

Injuries to the chest can occur in any sport and are not usually serious, though they can be worrisome. Chest injuries often result from a fall to the floor or playing field or from being hit by a ball, a piece of equipment, or another player's foot or hand.

Contusions (Bruises)

Because the muscles of the chest wall move with breathing and are attached to the shoulder and collarbone, bruises to those muscles can cause pain with breathing or movement of the arms. Rest and pain relievers are needed initially. A lingering problem can be secondary to stiffness and inflammation and may require nonsteroidal anti-inflammatories.

Bruised Breast and Nipples

These should be treated like muscle contusions. Sometimes a large black-and-blue mark remains over the breast, but this usually goes away on its own in 7 to 10 days. Use of a firm-fitting bra with some padding over the bruised area should provide adequate protection during participation in most sports.

Broken Rib

You should suspect a broken rib when an athlete experiences persistent, intense pain. The pain from a contusion can be intense, but the intensity does not persist. Athletes with broken ribs usually hold their chests with their hands and try not to breathe deeply because of the pain. The pain is usually localized and can be pointed to with one finger. An examination will reveal marked tenderness over one part of the rib. Examining ribs can be difficult, however, so do not hesitate to ask the team physician for help. If symptoms indicate a broken rib, have the athlete evaluated by a physician. Athletes with broken ribs can develop pneumothorax (collapsed lung) or bleeding in the lung. Because of this danger, they cannot compete in contact sports for two to three weeks. Broken ribs heal primarily with time and rest. Rib belts and taping of the chest are usually not recommended.

Chest Pain (without Trauma)

Keep in mind that weightlifting can strain chest muscles, and that athletes with colds or asthma can also suffer chest pain. Take a history, do an exam, and use common sense.

Abdomen (Stomach) Injuries

Injuries to the abdomen result from direct blows by feet, hands, or helmets and other pieces of equipment, as well as from contact with the playing surface. The muscles of the abdomen can also become sore or sustain partial tears from exercises such as "sit-ups." The major difficulty in dealing with injuries to the abdomen is deciding whether the injury involves only a muscle or whether it has affected the inner organs of the abdomen, such as the liver or the spleen.

Muscle injuries are treated with rest and pain relievers. Some torn muscles, such as those seen with a hip pointer, can take two to three weeks to heal. (A hip pointer is actually a tear in one of the abdominal muscles where it attaches to the top of the pelvis.) However, stomach muscle bruises or tears usually improve within hours.

Damage to internal organs should be suspected if any of the following occur:

- Pain becomes worse with time.
- Athlete becomes sick (i.e., nausea, vomiting, weakness).
- Athlete walks bent over, or lies down with legs drawn up toward stomach to relieve pain.
- Pain spreads to other areas of the abdomen.

Damage to internal organs such as the spleen or liver are accompanied by bleeding. This blood loss can be slow and may not cause symptoms initially, but with time the blood irritates the lining of the abdomen and produces the above symptoms.

When there is blood in the abdomen, the exam will reveal tenderness not only when you touch an area but also when you release your hand (rebound tenderness). **Rapid** physician evaluation is needed if you suspect an internal injury.

Injuries to the Testicles

A direct blow to a male athlete's groin produces severe pain, particularly if the testicles are bruised. The athlete usually drops to the playing surface, grasps his groin, and grimaces. Don't expect him to tell you where it hurts—the pain and embarrassment are too severe to allow much conversation.

The covering of the testicles is very tight and there is very little room for swelling, so any bruise is painful. The discomfort is usually temporary, however.

Bending the legs up toward the abdomen provides some initial relief. Athletes can often "walk it off" in three to four minutes and return to participation. Persistent mild discomfort can be treated with ice and a firm-fitting athletic supporter. If pain continues, a physician evaluation is indicated, as there may be an infection present.

Edward J. Shahady

10

Back Injuries

Approximately 5 percent of all athletic injuries occur to the back. Most of these are injuries to the muscles (see Fig. 10-1) and can be **acute**, resulting from either a blow or severe strain, or **chronic**, resulting from multiple small strains accumulated over a period of time. Injury to the spinal column and nerves is unusual. Weight training, football, and wrestling account for many acute back injuries. Chronic back pain can occur in any sport.

Acute Injuries

Upper-Back Bruises

Description

Bruises in this area are common to such sports as football and wrestling. They are not usually severe.

Symptoms

• Pain initially may be incapacitating, but it usually subsides quickly.

Exam

• Feel for tenderness over the involved muscles. The tenderness is ordinarily generalized. Pinpoint tenderness may indicate a broken rib or ribs.

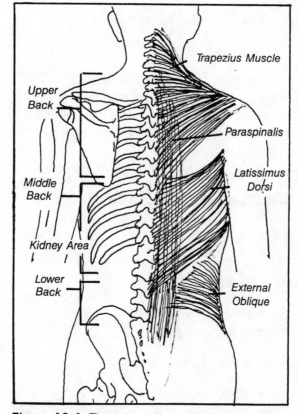

Figure 10-1. The regions and muscles of the back

Treatment

• Ice, rest, and nonsteroidal anti-inflammatories
• Stretching program designed specifically for the involved muscle groups (see exercises)

Mid-Back and Kidney Bruises

Description

These are similar to the upper-back bruises, but special attention must be given to bruises involving the kidneys. It is not easy to tell initially if the injury involves more than muscle.

Symptoms

• Pain in the mid-back, aggravated by movement.
• Pain may spread, involving the side or the abdomen (stomach).

Exam

• Palpate for tenderness over mid-back.

Treatment

• Ice, rest, and nonsteroidal anti-inflammatories.
• If the pain remains severe or spreads to involve the muscles on the side and front of the abdomen, the athlete should see a physician as this may indicate kidney damage.

Acute Lower-Back Pain

Description

Probably the most common causes of back pain in athletics are back strains and herniated (slipped) discs. These can both be caused by a direct blow to the back, but more often they result from a single movement that tears the muscle fibers.

Symptoms

• The athlete stands as straight as possible and usually holds the lower back with one hand while grimacing with pain (Fig. 10-2).
• The athlete often remembers the event that triggered the pain, which usually involves a twisting and forward movement of the body.
• The athlete may feel "a catch" in the lower back.
• Pain may extend into the buttocks or down one leg.
• The athlete has trouble getting up from a chair.
• Reaching down to remove shoes aggravates the pain.

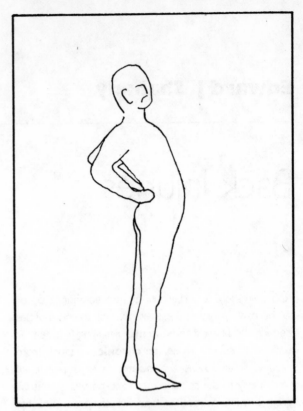

Figure 10-2. Typical back-pain posture

Exam

• Measure the degree of forward, backward, and lateral flexion (Fig. 10-3). Limitation in one or more of these movements is common if the back is injured.
• Perform the **straight leg raising test** (Fig. 10-4). This tests the tightness of the hamstring as well as indicating pressure on the nerves from a disc. Test both legs. A positive test produces pain in the back. Tightness causes pain in the hamstring muscles.
• Ask the athlete to walk on toes, then heels. If the heels or toes cannot be kept elevated for four to five steps, there is some weakness. Weakness in one leg may be due to pressure on a nerve from a disc and indicates the need for physician referral.

Treatment

• Ice and nonsteroidal anti-inflammatories.
• Some injuries may require 2 to 3 days of bed rest.
• Exercises can help decrease muscle spasms and strengthen the back muscles. Many athletes find that back pain remains for life but can be controlled with common sense and proper exercises.

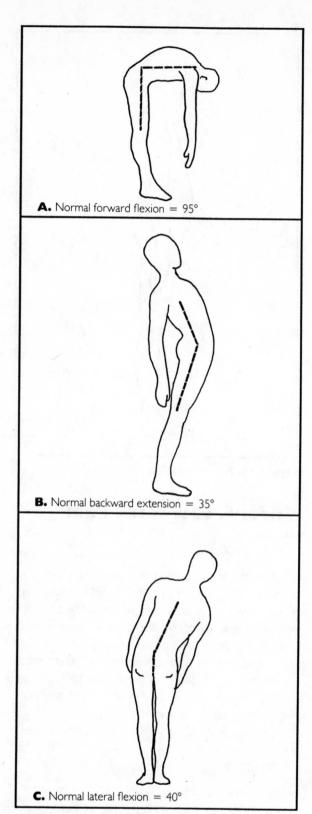

A. Normal forward flexion = 95°

B. Normal backward extension = 35°

C. Normal lateral flexion = 40°

Figure 10-3. Back flexion

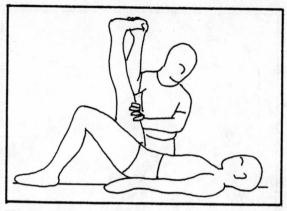

Figure 10-4. Straight leg raising test

Prevention

Follow guidelines for sleeping, sitting, standing, and lifting (see below).

Chronic Injuries

Chronic Pain in the Mid-Back

Description

Recurrent back pain that is aggravated by activity and bending can be caused by a problem known as **Scheuermann's disease**. The pain is usually located at the mid-back where the thoracic vertebrae meet the lumbar vertebrae (Fig. 10-5). This problem is unique to adolescents between 14 and 18 years of age. These patients also begin to develop rounding of the upper back.

Symptoms

• Pain located in the mid-back, aggravated by activity and bending.

Exam

• Look for rounding of the back.

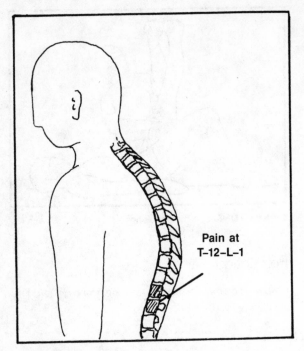

Figure 10-5. Scheuermann's disease

Pain at
T–12–L–1

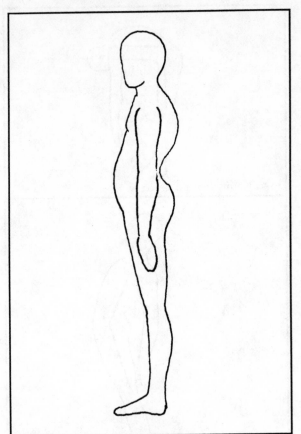

Figure 10-7. Lumbar lordosis

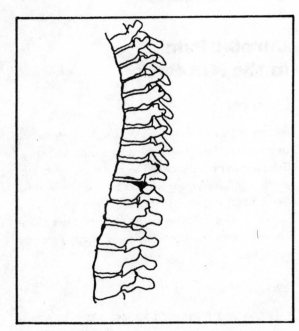

Figure 10-6. Spondylolysis

Chronic Low-Back Pain

Description

Most instances of chronic low-back pain are due to weak muscles and respond to exercise. However, chronic low-back pain can also be caused by an entity known as **spondylolysis**. Spondylolysis is considered a stress fracture of one of the bones in the back (Fig. 10-6) and requires further treatment. It occurs most frequently in such sports as gymnastics, football, and weight training. Teenage athletes who complain of persistent low-back pain should be taken seriously, as spondylolysis is the cause in 30 percent of these cases.

Symptoms

- Tenderness over the back.
- An athlete with spondylolysis has a characteristic stance due to tight hamstring muscles and weak abdominal muscles, which increase lumbar lordosis (curved spine) (Fig. 10-7).

Treatment

- Rest.
- Since diagnosis is made with the aid of an X ray, any athlete who exhibits symptoms of this nature should be evaluated by a physician.

- An athlete with spondylolysis experiences a gradual pain at the onset, usually described as stiffness in the lower back and upper buttocks.
- The pain is usually worse during and immediately following an athletic event. In the early stages of the disease, the pain goes away after the event, but as the disease develops, the pain persists throughout waking hours.

Exam

- Palpate for tenderness over the back. Do not be misled if this fails to reproduce the pain.
- Perform the same tests explained under "Acute Lower-Back Pain." Look for hamstring tightness but no muscle weakness.

Treatment

- Back exercises to strengthen abdominal muscles and increase flexibility of hamstring muscles. These must be performed faithfully in order to have any real effect.

- If symptoms indicate spondylolysis, refer the athlete to a physician.
- A back brace may be necessary. The exercises and the brace are geared toward decreasing curvature in the back.

Prevention

Include strengthening and flexibility exercises designed for the back and related areas in the athlete's routine strengthening program. Emphasize proper technique in all sports, particularly in weight training. Many back injuries can be avoided if proper techniques are taught and consistently followed.

Exercises for Low-Back Pain

Back Stretch

• Lie on back with arms above head and knees bent. Move one knee as far as possible toward chest while straightening the other leg. Return to original position with both knees bent, and repeat the movement, alternating legs (Fig. 10-8).

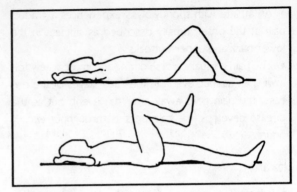

Figure 10-8

Back Stretch

• Lie on back with a small pillow under head, arms at sides and knees bent. Bring knees up to chest, and then pull knees toward chest with arms. Hold for a count of ten, keeping knees together and shoulders flat on the mat, then return to beginning position. Repeat 3 times. Relax and repeat the exercise (Fig. 10-9).

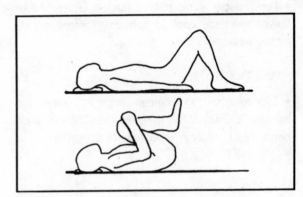

Figure 10-9

Back Stretch

• Lie on back with arms above head and knees bent. Tighten lower abdomen and buttock muscles at the same time, flattening back against the mat. Relax and repeat the exercise (Fig. 10-10).

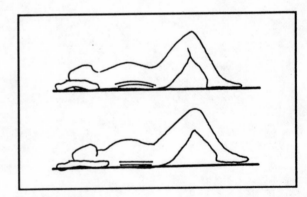

Figure 10-10

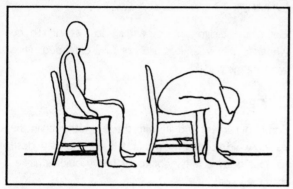

Figure 10-11

Abdomen Curls

• Sit on a hard chair with arms loosely at sides. Let body drop forward until head is between knees. Pull body back up into a sitting position while tightening abdominal muscles. Relax and repeat the exercise (Fig. 10-11).

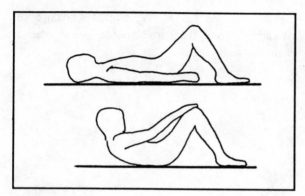

Figure 10-12

Abdomen Curls

• See Figure 10-12.

NOTE: All exercises should be done 30 times each.

Taking Care of the Back

Sitting

Use a hard chair and put spine up against it; try to keep one or both knees higher than hips (a small stool is helpful here). For short rest periods, a contour chair offers excellent support.

Standing

Try to stand with lower back straight. When standing, use a footrest to help relieve swayback. Never lean forward without bending knees. **Women take note**: Shoes with moderate heels strain the back less than those with high heels. Avoid platform shoes.

Sleeping

Sleep on a firm mattress. If your mattress is soft, put a bedboard (¾" plywood) under it. Do not sleep on your stomach. If you sleep on your back, put a pillow under your knees. If you sleep on your side, keep your legs bent at the knees and at the hips.

Driving

Get a hard seat for your car and sit close enough to the wheel so that your legs are not fully extended while working the pedals.

Lifting

Bend your knees and lift with the legs rather than the back. Avoid sudden movements. Keep the load close to your body and try not to lift heavy objects higher than the waist.

Exercise

Get regular exercise (walking, swimming, etc.) once backache is gone. But start slowly to give muscles a chance to warm up.

Stanley R. Watson

Shoulder Injuries

Up to 13 percent of all athletic injuries involve the shoulder. Shoulder injuries usually result from a direct blow, a forceful strain, or from highly repetitive motions that produce overuse injuries. Consequently, such sports as swimming, baseball, volleyball, football, and wrestling have the highest risk of shoulder injury.

The shoulder's three major bones are the **clavicle** (collarbone), the **scapula** (shoulder blade), and the **humerus** (upper armbone). The collarbone attaches at one end to the **sternum**, or breastbone, and at the other end to the **acromion process**, the tip of the shoulder (Fig. 11-1). The humerus fits into the scapula like a ball on a shallow saucer and is held in place by a cuff of four muscles known as the **rotator cuff**. These muscles consist of the **supraspinatus**, **infraspinatus**, **teres minor**, and **subscapularis** (Fig. 11-2). The shoulder also consists of various ligaments that connect portions of the bones together and strengthen the joints, such as the **acromioclavicular**, **coracoclavicular**, and **coracoacromial** ligaments (Fig. 11-3).

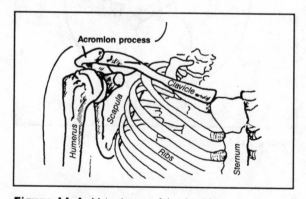

Figure 11-1. Major bones of the shoulder

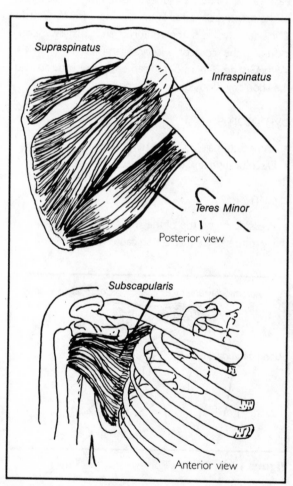

Figure 11-2. Muscles of the rotator cuff

Shoulder Separation

(A/C Separation)

Description

Shoulder separations, also known as **acromioclavicular (A/C) separations**, usually result from a direct blow to the shoulder and are often confused with dislocations, though the two injuries are actually quite dissimilar. A separation is a rupture of the ligaments connecting the collarbone and the acromion process, whereas a dislocation involves the displacement of the humerus from the scapula. There are three major grades of shoulder separations, and it is important to distinguish between the grades, as the treatment for each varies. **Grade 1** injuries involve only a slight sprain of the acromioclavicular ligaments (Fig. 11-4A). **Grade 2** injuries involve some ruptured and torn ligaments, including the coracoclavicular ligaments (Fig. 11-4B). With **Grade 3** injuries, all ligaments are ruptured and the shoulder is obviously deformed (Fig. 11-4C).

Symptoms

- Immediate pain (Fig. 11-5)
- Discoloration and deformity in severe cases

Exam

- Press down on top of the shoulder or pull down on the arm to see if either action causes pain.

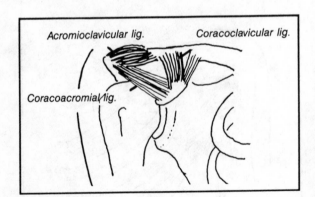

Figure 11-3. Shoulder ligaments

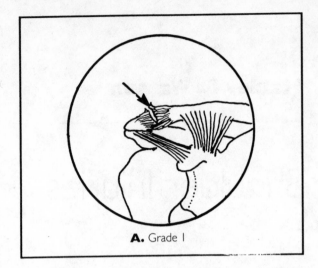

A. Grade 1

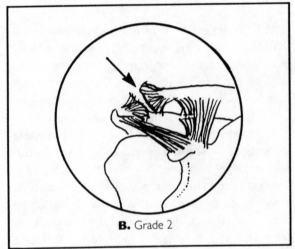

B. Grade 2

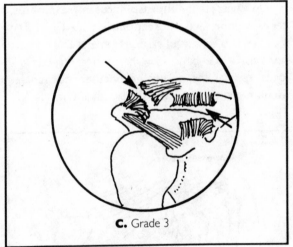

C. Grade 3

Figure 11-4. Shoulder separations

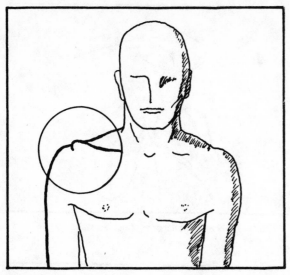

Figure 11-5. Location of pain with shoulder separation

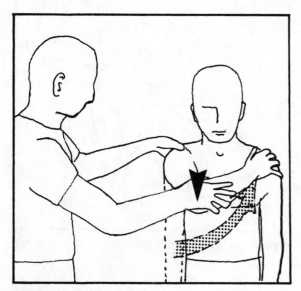

Figure 11-6. "Crossover" test

• See if the athlete experiences pain when attempting to move the shoulder.
• Have the athlete perform the "crossover" test (Fig. 11-6) by touching the top of the uninjured shoulder with the hand of the injured one. Push down on the elbow while the athlete resists the movement. With Grade 1 injuries, the athlete experiences pain but can resist movement. With Grade 2 injuries, the pain is too severe to allow resistance. With Grade 3 injuries, severe pain makes it impossible for the athlete to touch the top of the uninjured shoulder with the hand of the injured arm.

Treatment

• Apply ice immediately.
• Place the injured arm in a sling and refer the athlete to a physician.

Rehabilitation

• Athletes with a mild (Grade 1) separation should be able to begin shoulder-strengthening exercises as soon as they no longer have pain at rest (within 2 to 7 days). These athletes may return to competition when they feel no pain even in response to applied pressure.
• A moderate (Grade 2) injury usually requires 10 to 14 days in a sling before strengthening exercises can begin. Recovery usually takes 14 to 21 days.
• A severe shoulder separation (Grade 3) may require surgery and prolonged rehabilitation.

Shoulder Dislocation

Description

A shallow socket affords the shoulder a wide range of motion but does little to prevent the humerus from slipping out. Instead, the rotator cuff muscles, along with cartilage and ligaments, provide the needed stability. However, sufficient impact can force the humerus outside of the socket or glenoid rim. If the humerus pops out and stays out, the injury is called a **dislocation**. If the humeral head comes out of its socket but spontaneously relocates, it is called a subluxation (see the following section). When the humerus dislocates, it can do so in any one of three directions:

1. A **forward (anterior) dislocation** (Fig. 11-7) is the most common type of shoulder dislocation. Forward dislocations commonly occur as a result of arm tackling in football or when a player's shot is blocked forcefully in volleyball or basketball.

2. A **backward (posterior) dislocation** (Fig. 11-8) can be caused by a direct blow to the front of the shoulder or by falling on an outstretched elbow when the fingers are turned in toward the body.

3. A **downward (inferior) dislocation** (Fig. 11-9) is caused by a blow to the top of the shoulder when the arm is stretched out to the side.

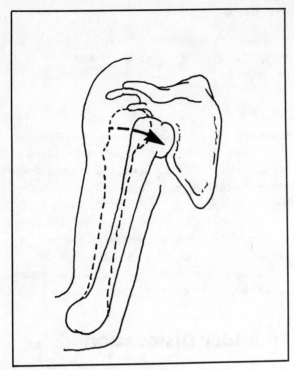

Figure 11-7. Forward (anterior) dislocation

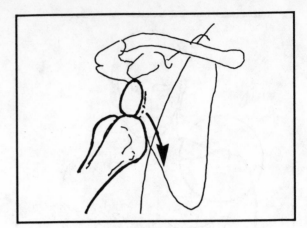

Figure 11-9. Downward (inferior) dislocation

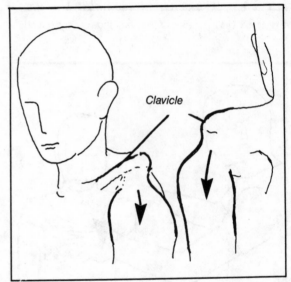

Clavicle

Figure 11-10. Forward (anterior) dislocation viewed from front and back

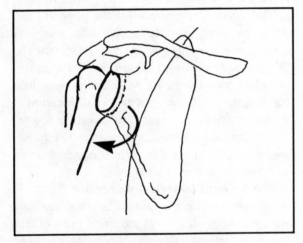

Figure 11-8. Backward (posterior) dislocation

Symptoms

- The athlete will feel severe pain.
- He or she may claim to have heard the shoulder pop and will resist moving the injured arm.

Exam

- Have the athlete attempt to rotate the arm or perform the "crossover" test (see Fig. 11-6). If the shoulder has been dislocated, the athlete will be unable to do either.
- Compare the injured shoulder with the uninjured one. **A dislocated shoulder appears square rather than rounded** (Fig. 11-10).

Treatment

- Place ice on the shoulder, keeping the arm in the most comfortable position for the athlete. **Do not attempt to pop the shoulder back in place**.
- The athlete should see a physician as soon as possible. The longer the shoulder stays dislocated, the more difficult it is to relocate.

Rehabilitation

• The athlete will be sidelined for 6 to 12 weeks but should begin a program of shoulder-strengthening exercises within the first few weeks after the injury occurs. A physical therapist usually initiates this program, but **coaches and trainers play a major role** in seeing that the athlete consistently adheres to the program during rehabilitation.

Shoulder Subluxation

(Swimmer's Shoulder)

Description

Subluxations occur when the humerus pops out of its socket but then spontaneously relocates, often due to a forceful twisting backward as the arm is raised overhead or to the side. Although subluxation is not as serious as dislocation, the unnatural movement of the bone damages muscles and ligaments. Posterior subluxations frequently afflict athletes who repeatedly use an overhand motion, particularly swimmers and baseball and tennis players. Subluxations are also fairly common in football, volleyball, and wrestling.

Symptoms

• Sudden pain; **the arm goes "dead" for a few moments**. (This may happen several times before an athlete brings it to anyone's attention.)

Exam

• Examine for subluxation in all directions (anterior, posterior, or inferior).
• The apprehension or "bye-bye" test (Fig. 11-11) checks anterior stability. Stand behind the athlete and place forward pressure on the humerus while the athlete rotates the humerus using a hand-waving movement.
• Testing for the other subluxations (Figs. 11-12, 11-13) involves placing backward or downward pressure on the humerus while the athlete is lying on a table. Compare the amount of movement in the injured shoulder with that on the uninjured side.

Treatment

• Rest, ice, and pain medication

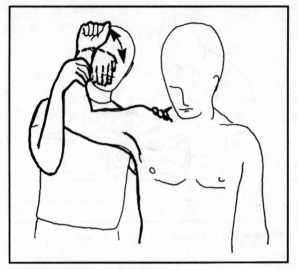

Figure 11-11. Apprehension or "bye-bye" test for anterior subluxation

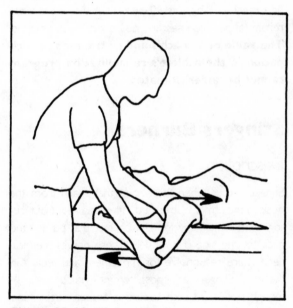

Figure 11-12. Inferior subluxation test

Rehabilitation

• Rehabilitation should begin after acute discomfort subsides. Exercises described in Figures 11-27, 11-28, 11-29, and 11-30 should be initiated and continued for at least 3 months. The athlete may return to competition when the apprehension tests elicit no pain.
• Athletes who experience **recurrent subluxations** should see a physician and give serious consideration either to discontinuing the sport or to utilizing a harness to reduce the risk of subluxations.

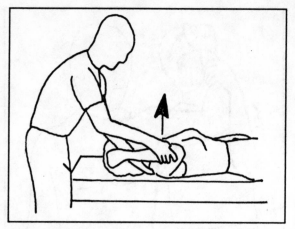

Figure 11-13. Posterior subluxation test

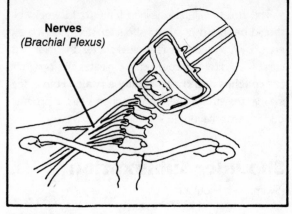

Figure 11-14. Neck stinger

Prevention

• The incidence of recurrent dislocation and subluxation can be as high as 80 percent if the appropriate rehabilitation exercises are not diligently performed. **The value of a coach's and/or trainer's participation in the athlete's rehabilitation program cannot be underestimated.**

Stingers/Burners

Description

Stingers occur when the nerves that reach from the neck to the arm are stretched, often as a result of tackling, blocking, or any forceful contact that pushes the neck to one side (Fig. 11-14). These nerves (cervical nerves) are responsible for movement and feeling in the arm. Stingers are most common in football, although players in such sports as soccer, rugby, and basketball are also at risk. It is important to note that although the injury actually occurs in the neck, the symptoms appear in the shoulder and arm.

Symptoms

• Severe pain in the shoulder, with an electric sensation shooting down the arm. **The pain and electric sensation of a stinger can frighten an athlete,** who may lie on the ground writhing in pain or come running to the sideline holding the injured arm and grimacing.

Exam

• There may be extreme tenderness over the upper portion of the humerus that usually subsides within one hour. The initial examination must rule out other causes of shoulder pain, such as a broken collarbone or a dislocated or separated shoulder.
• **Test for the strength of the various shoulder muscles** (Figs. 11-15, 11-16, 11-17). With stingers, one or more muscles can be weakened.

Treatment

• Place the arm in a comfortable position and apply ice to painful areas. Some stingers are mild and do not seriously limit activity.

Rehabilitation

• With the cessation of pain and the return of muscular strength, the athlete should be able to return to competition. However, some stingers can be quite disabling and may take up to a year to heal. If muscle strength has not returned in 24 hours, the athlete should be evaluated by a physician.
• Strengthening the weakened muscles through exercise is extremely important to recovery. **Athletes recovering from stingers are more susceptible to shoulder subluxation if the rotator cuff and deltoid muscles remain weak.**

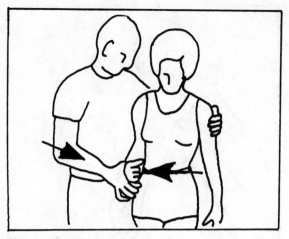

Figure 11-15. Test for strength of external rotators (infraspinatus and teres minor)

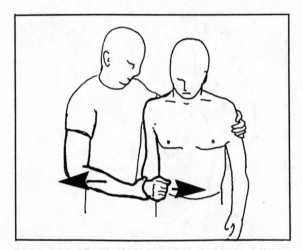

Figure 11-16. Test for strength of internal rotators (subscapularis)

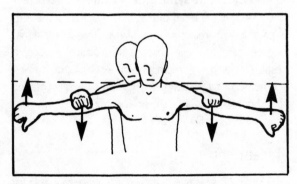

Figure 11-17. Test for strength of supraspinatus

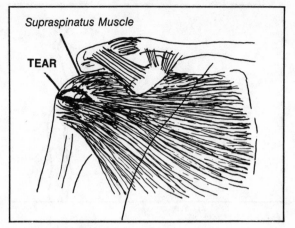

Figure 11-18. Rotator cuff tear

Prevention

Athletes with recurrent stingers may benefit from wearing a neck collar. These collars are especially helpful to athletes with long necks who are more susceptible to stingers.

Rotator Cuff Injuries

Description

The four muscles comprising the rotator cuff (supraspinatus, infraspinatus, teres minor, and subscapularis), form a cuff over the humeral head. These muscles stabilize the shoulder and are responsible for helping the shoulder rotate and lifting the arm out from the body. There are two basic types of rotator cuff injuries. One is the **rotator cuff tear** (Fig. 11-18), which is fairly uncommon. A tear involves the supraspinatus muscle and causes the athlete to have difficulty abducting (lifting) the arm. Tears cause pain during athletic activity and significant discomfort at night. The second, and the most common, type of rotator cuff injury is the **impingement syndrome**. This occurs when the supraspinatus muscle is impinged (squeezed) between the ligaments and the bones and becomes swollen; over time the muscle becomes inflamed, weakens, and may rupture. There are five stages to the impingement syndrome. Young athletes will experience only the earlier stages (i.e., swelling and inflammation). Rupture does not usually occur until an athlete is aged 40 to 50, after many years of using the shoulder for throwing or other overhand motions. Although young athletes seldom ex-

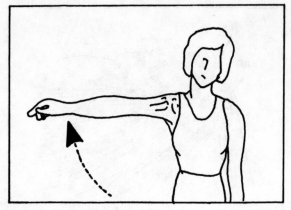

A. Athlete raises arm.

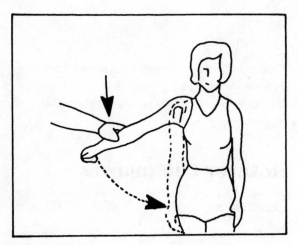

B. Arm drops after being tapped gently.

Figure 11-19. Drop-arm test

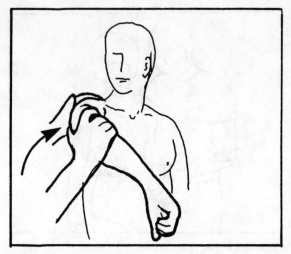

Figure 11-20. Impingement test (internal rotation)

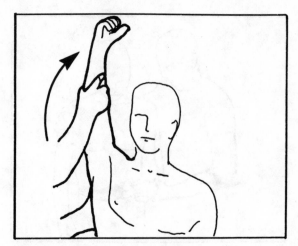

Figure 11-21. Impingement test (forward flexion)

perience the latter stages of impingement, recognizing and treating the early stages is crucial in halting progression to the latter stages. Rotator cuff tears and the impingement syndrome are both overuse injuries caused by repetitive arm movements such as throwing.

Symptoms

• The athlete complains of discomfort in the shoulder, similar to that of a toothache, that appears after the athletic endeavor.

Exam

• **Tears**. The "drop-arm" test detects tears in the supraspinatus muscle. Have the athlete lift his or her arm to a 90-degree angle (Fig. 11-19A). A gentle tap should then cause the arm to drop to the athlete's side (Fig. 11-19B).

• **Impingement syndrome**. Palpation reveals tenderness over the head of the humerus; raising the arm is painful, with maximum pain when the arm is at 90 degrees; and an impingement test produces a positive result (elicits pain). Impingement tests include flexing the humerus to 90 degrees and then internally rotating the shoulder (Fig. 11-20), or forcibly flexing the humerus forward (Fig. 11-21).

Treatment

• The key is selective rest. The activity responsible for causing impingement must be decreased or completely stopped until the activity produces no pain and strength is normal.

Rehabilitation

• A program of stretching and strengthening exercises for rotator cuff muscles is vital once the athlete feels ready to resume competition.
• It also helps for the athlete to apply heat prior to activity and ice immediately following and to use non-steroidal anti-inflammatories.

Prevention

Teaching athletes who are at risk for rotator cuff injuries specific techniques for decreasing impingement stress can help decrease the incidence of the syndrome. Stretching exercises for the rotator cuff should be employed before every practice. Throwing short distances at a slower speed for 10 to 20 minutes or swimming easy distances for 10 minutes before sprinting are two examples of warm-ups that help decrease impingement.

Sore Arm

Description

A sore arm, the most common overuse injury in high school athletics, results when muscles do not get enough blood to handle the strain placed on them due to misuse or improper warm-up.

Symptoms

• Pain in any area of the shoulder may be intense and throbbing shortly after exercise but decreases quickly with rest.

Exam

• Compare the injured shoulder to the uninjured one, checking for swelling, pain, and deformity.
• Gently palpate to locate the area that hurts the most. Make sure the athlete can move the shoulder in all directions.

Treatment

• The athlete should undergo P-R-I-C-E for 24 to 48 hours. **An athlete should never try to "throw through" a sore arm**, as this can only cause worse damage.

Rehabilitation

• After a few days of rest, the athlete can *gradually* begin using the shoulder. Begin the recovery sequence by stretching, followed by warm-up exercises and gentle use of the shoulder, before proceeding to moderate and full use. If pain recurs at any point, the athlete should stop immediately and apply ice for 24 hours before beginning the recovery sequence again.

Broken Collarbone

Description

A broken collarbone, or fractured clavicle, usually occurs when the collarbone receives a direct blow of considerable force. In younger athletes, a forceful hit on the side of the shoulder can cause a fracture.

Symptoms

• Pain and possible bruising or swelling anywhere along the length of the collarbone, usually focused in the middle of the bone. Swelling usually starts within 6 hours.
• The athlete may feel the bones rubbing together, and the injured shoulder may droop forward or downward.
• **All motion is painful**.

Exam

• Check for the above symptoms of a break.
• Gently press around the painful area; it may be possible to feel the broken ends of the bone.

Treatment

• Apply ice immediately and put the arm in a sling. X rays are necessary to determine if a break has actually occurred.

Rehabilitation

• The arm should remain in a sling for 3 to 4 weeks. Healing takes 6 to 8 weeks, and an exercise program to strengthen the shoulder can begin once the bones have healed.

Shoulder Exercises

Stretching the Rotator Cuff

Before beginning any other exercises, stretch the capsule around the shoulder joint by lying on a table with a one- or two-pound weight in your hand and with your shoulder extending over the table edge.

Figures 11-22, 11-23, and 11-24 show three different positions for stretching the rotator cuff. In Figure 11-22 the shoulder is at 90 degrees and in Figure 11-23 at 135 degrees. In Figure 11-24 the arm extends over the head. Allow the weight to pull your arm down into each of these positions. Hold the stretch for 10 to 12 seconds, then repeat 5 to 8 times.

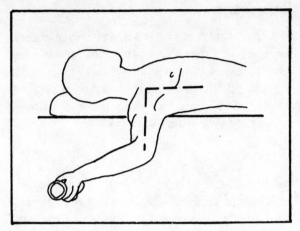

Figure 11-22. Rotator cuff stretch—90°

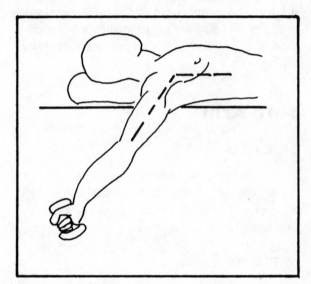

Figure 11-23. Rotator cuff stretch—135°

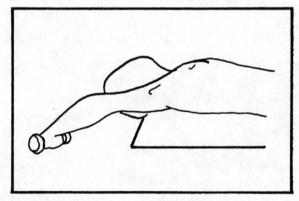

Figure 11-24. Rotator cuff stretch with arm overhead

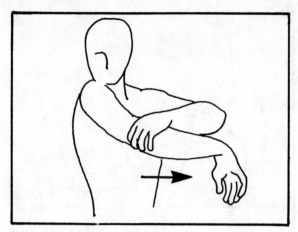

Figure 11-25. Posterior cuff stretch

Do the next two stretches without a weight. Stretch the posterior cuff by pulling your arm across in front of your body (Fig. 11-25). Stretch the inferior cuff by reaching overhead and gently pulling on your elbow with the opposite hand (Fig. 11-26). Hold both stretches for 10 to 12 seconds and repeat 5 to 8 times. Do all of the stretches two times daily.

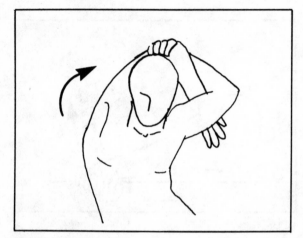

Figure 11-26. Inferior cuff stretch

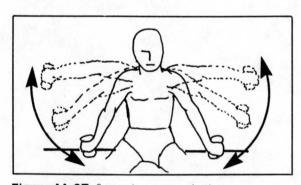

Figure 11-27. Supraspinatus strengthening

Shoulder Strengthening

These exercises should focus on specific muscles. Start with just a few pounds of weight and gradually increase.

Supraspinatus Muscle

• Do this exercise with the elbow straight and the thumb turned toward the floor. Slowly raise your arm to shoulder level but no higher (Fig. 11-27). Hold for 5 seconds and lower slowly.

External Rotation (Infraspinatus and Teres Minor)

• Lie on your side with your upper elbow against your ribs and raise the weight as high as possible without lifting your elbow. Hold 5 seconds, then lower slowly (Fig. 11-28A).

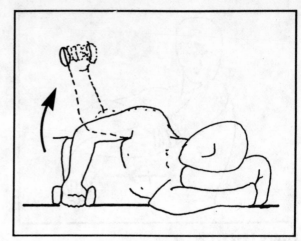

A. External rotation

Internal Rotation (Subscapularis)

• Lie on your back with your arm next to your side and bent at the elbow. Raise the weight and hold it for 5 seconds, then lower slowly (Fig. 11-28B).

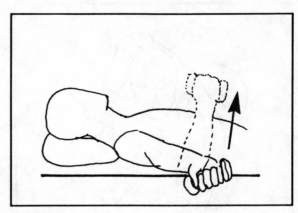

B. Internal rotation

Figure 11-28. Shoulder rotations

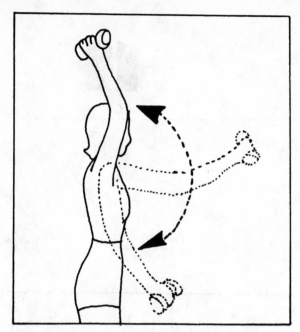

Figure 11-29. Shoulder flexion

Shoulder Flexion (Deltoid)

• Stand with your arm at your side and, keeping the elbow straight, raise the weight to an overhead position. Hold 5 seconds and lower it again slowly (Fig. 11-29).

Shoulder Abduction (Deltoid)

• The central deltoid is one of the most powerful muscles in the shoulder. Lift the weight from your side to a 90-degree angle and then overhead (Fig. 11-30). Note the position of the hand with the thumb pointed upward, in contrast to the supraspinatus exercise in which the thumb points down.

NOTE: All of these shoulder exercises should be done every day. Begin by doing two sets of 10 repetitions each, using a one- or two-pound weight. You can gradually increase the weight, but do not cause soreness.

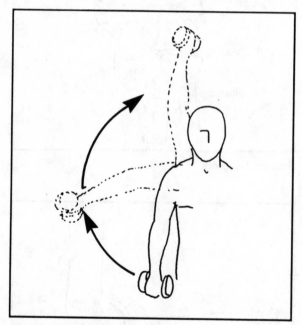

Figure 11-30. Shoulder abduction

John E. Blake

12

Elbow Injuries

Athletes are most vulnerable to elbow injuries when participating in contact sports or sports requiring extensive throwing. Baseball, tennis, wrestling, gymnastics, and some field events in track have the highest risk of elbow injuries. Bruises (contusions) to soft tissue around the elbow are common in all sports. Overuse injuries to the elbow are particularly common in baseball, tennis, and golf.

The elbow works like a hinge, performing a variety of motions such as bending (flexion) and straightening (extension) of the forearm and rotational movements (supination and pronation) at the elbow, allowing the hand to turn palm up and palm down. The elbow joint is formed by the upper armbone, or humerus, and the two forearm bones, the radius and the ulna (Fig. 12-1). Important muscles include the elbow flexors (biceps and brachialis) and extensors (triceps) and the wrist extensors and flexors (Figs. 12-2, 12-3).

Elbow Sprain
(Hyperextended Elbow)

Description

Elbow sprains occur when the arm is straightened further than the elbow allows (hyperextension) usually as the result either of a fall on the outstretched hand or of a blow received on the outside of the elbow when the arm is straight and the hand firmly placed on a hard surface (Fig. 12-4).

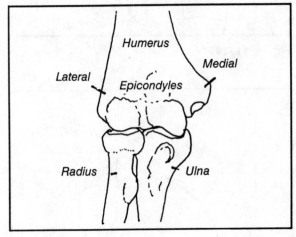

Anterior (front) view

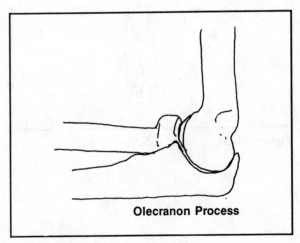

Lateral (side) view

Figure 12-1. Bones of the elbow

64

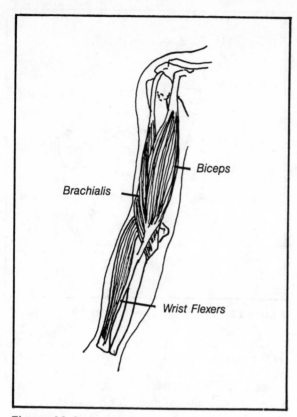

Figure 12-2. Anterior (front) view of arm

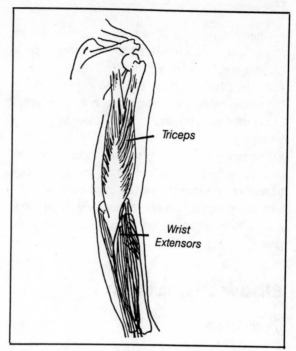

Figure 12-3. Posterior (back) view of arm

Symptoms

• Moderate pain that gradually intensifies as a result of swelling.
• Specific pain sites may include the inside (medial) and front (anterior) of the elbow.
• The athlete complains of weakness in the arm.

Exam

• Observe the elbow for signs of swelling and deformity.
• Feel (palpate) to locate the painful sites.
• Ask the athlete to straighten/bend the elbow to check for limited movement. The athlete will not allow the arm to be completely straightened (full extension).

Treatment

• Apply ice immediately.
• Utilize a sling to reduce pain and stress to the elbow.
• Give nonsteroidal anti-inflammatories to help pain and relieve swelling.
• Refer the athlete to a physician.

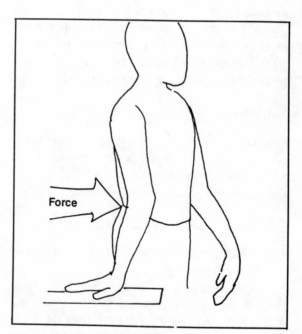

Figure 12-4. Hyperextended elbow

Rehabilitation

• After 4 days, range of motion will increase and the athlete should be encouraged to move the elbow as much as possible without pain.

• As the athlete gradually begins to regain motion in the elbow, he or she should exercise the joint until it regains full mobility and strength (approximately 4 weeks).

• The timing of the athlete's return to full activity will depend on the severity of the sprain. Taping the elbow to restrict full extension may enable the athlete to return earlier and still prevent reinjury (Fig. 12-5). However, a fully recovered and unrestricted elbow is the goal.

Elbow Dislocation

Description

Elbow dislocations usually result from falling on an outstretched hand with the elbow extended, but they can also occur when the elbow is twisted while in a bent (flexed) position. A direct blow to the back (posterior) or outer (lateral) side of the elbow while the hand is planted can cause a dislocation if the force is significantly greater than the resistance of the elbow joint.

Symptoms

• Severe pain and disability; the athlete is unable to put weight on the hand or move the arm normally.

• The forearm may become numb.

• The arm is usually flexed to 45 degrees.

Exam

• Check for a pulse at the wrist. No pulse indicates an arm-threatening emergency.

• Stroke and/or prick the forearm, hand, and fingers to check for sensation.

• **DO NOT ATTEMPT TO POP (RELOCATE) THE ELBOW BACK INTO THE JOINT!**

• The most distinct aspect of dislocation is obvious deformity. The forearm (radius and/or ulna) will be displaced forward, backward, or laterally. Most common is the backward dislocation of the forearm, wherein the injured arm appears shorter than the uninjured arm and the tip of the elbow (olecranon) appears to be larger and set further back (Fig. 12-6).

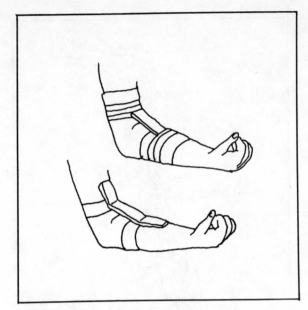

Figure 12-5. Elbow extension restriction taping

Treatment

• Apply ice with a pressure bandage, place the arm in a sling, and refer the athlete to a physician.

Rehabilitation

• During the period of immobilization (usually 3 to 4 weeks), the athlete should perform hand-gripping and shoulder exercises.

• After the initial healing period, the athlete should begin passive exercises to regain motion in the elbow, increasing gradually to active exercises.

Elbow Fractures

Description

Elbow fractures are usually caused by falling on the outstretched hand or by a direct blow to the elbow. Younger athletes are more vulnerable to this type of injury than adults. Any of the bones in the elbow may be affected. Fractures often occur in conjunction with the hyperextended (sprained) elbow and the dislocated elbow.

Symptoms

• There may not be a visible deformity, but swelling, pain, and muscle spasm are usually evident.

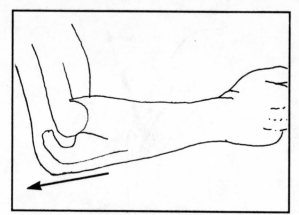

Figure 12-6. Backward (posterior) dislocation

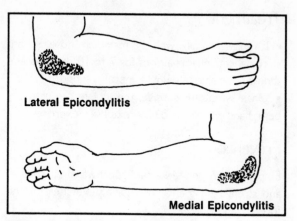

Figure 12-7. Locations of tennis elbow pain

Exam

• Same as for dislocations

Treatment

• Apply ice and mild pressure immediately, place the arm in a sling, and refer the athlete to a physician.

Rehabilitation

• Same as for dislocations

Tennis Elbow

Description

Tennis elbow, or **epicondylitis**, is a chronic condition caused by repeated rotation and forced extension of the forearm. It is also called "pitcher's elbow" or "golfer's elbow," depending on the sport involved. Injuries labeled "tennis elbow" are actually muscle tears, sprains to ligaments, or tendinitis in the elbow, but all begin because of (1) repetitive stress to the elbow; (2) improper technique; (3) poor warm-up; (4) poor conditioning of the arm (elbow); or (5) putting excessive stress on the elbow at an early age.

Symptoms

• Pain on the outside (lateral) or inside (medial) part of the elbow (Fig. 12-7).
• Pain may radiate down the arm.
• Active movements of the forearm and elbow cause pain.

Exam

• Have the athlete make a fist and cock the wrist. Try to force the wrist down while the athlete forces it up (Fig. 12-8A). Severe pain over the lateral epicondyle (see Fig. 12-7) indicates lateral tennis elbow.
• To check for medial tennis elbow, resist as the athlete pushes the fist down (Fig. 12-8B). Pain should occur over the medial epicondyle.

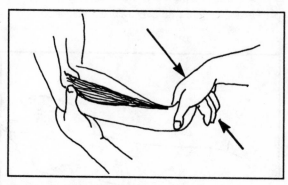

A. Lateral epicondylitis test

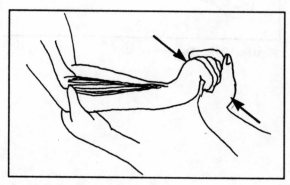

B. Medial epicondylitis test

Figure 12-8. Tests for tennis elbow

Treatment

• Ice massage daily, with the maximum dose of non-steroidal anti-inflammatories for 7 to 10 days. Athlete should not participate until symptoms subside.
• Once symptoms subside, the athlete can gradually begin hand-gripping and hand-extension exercises.

Prevention

Emphasize proper technique, good warm-up routine, and strengthening and conditioning exercises for the forearm and elbow.

Little League Elbow

This refers to elbow pain in athletes whose bones are still growing (usually those between ages ten and fourteen, but occasionally up to fifteen or sixteen). A future loss of strength in the arm, or even the use of it, are serious possibilities if the condition goes untreated. Any sign of persistent elbow pain deserves physician evaluation. Chronic elbow pain can afflict not only pitchers and catchers in Little League baseball, but also tennis players and golfers who overtrain at a young age.

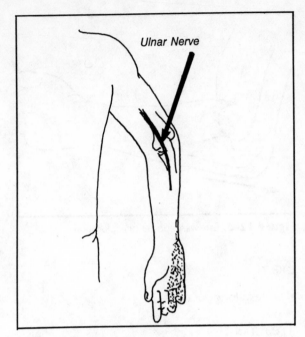

Figure 12-10. Ulnar nerve

Elbow Bruises

Description

The back, or tip, of the elbow is particularly vulnerable to blows that result in bruising. Keep in mind that elbow bruises can have possible complications such as fracture, synovitis, or olecranon bursitis.

Symptoms

• Pain and swelling (sometimes rapid)

Exam

• Carefully check for the location of point tenderness.
• Refer an athlete with severe pain over a bony area of the elbow to a physician.

Treatment

• P-R-I-C-E and nonsteroidal anti-inflammatories

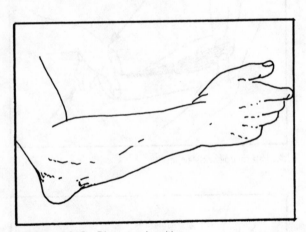

Figure 12-9. Olecranon bursitis

Olecranon Bursitis

Description

The tip of the elbow (ulna) is called the **olecranon** and has soft tissue covering it to reduce friction and stress.

This soft tissue is called the **bursa** (olecranon bursa). When it receives a blow, the bursa can become very swollen and inflamed (Fig. 12-9).

Symptoms

- Immediate pain with swelling.
- Occasionally there is spontaneous swelling without pain.
- The injury site often feels hot.

Exam

- Careful palpation reveals soft, swollen tissue.

Treatment

- For acute olecranon bursitis, apply ice with pressure from a wrap.
- If swelling is chronic, the elbow needs to be drained (aspirated) by a doctor.
- The elbow should be well padded before the athlete returns to play.

NOTE: This injury is annoying but seldom serious.

Ulnar Nerve ("Funny Bone") Injuries

Description

The back of the elbow commonly receives blows that send a shooting pain down the arm into the hand (Fig. 12-10). Athletes call this hitting the "funny bone." It is not a serious injury unless an athlete has recurrent problems with elbow pain, which can be a sign of the nerve being trapped or pinched (impinged).

Symptoms

- The athlete complains of a burning and tingling sensation in the fourth and fifth fingers.

Treatment

- Protect the elbow with padding without putting pressure on the nerve.
- Padding does nothing for chronic nerve injuries. In this case, the athlete needs to see a physician.

Elbow Exercises

Elbow Flexion/Biceps Curl

With a one- to two-pound weight in your hand, hold your elbow close to your side and lift the weight slowly in front of you (Fig. 12-11). Return arm to complete extension.

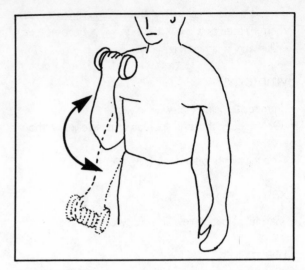

Figure 12-11

Triceps Exercise

With a one- or two-pound weight in your hand, sit or stand with your elbow bent and the hand dropped back behind your head; support the arm with your opposite hand (Fig. 12-12). Raise the bent arm upward until straight and lower slowly.

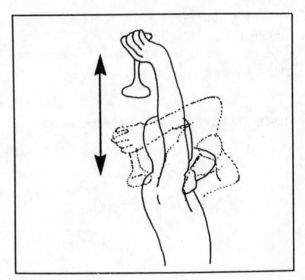

Figure 12-12

Towel Twist

Hold a towel between your hands. Twist the towel backward and forward between your hands (Fig. 12-13).

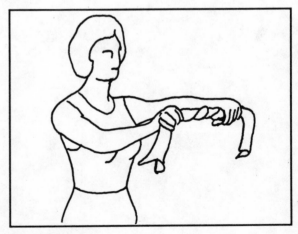

Figure 12-13

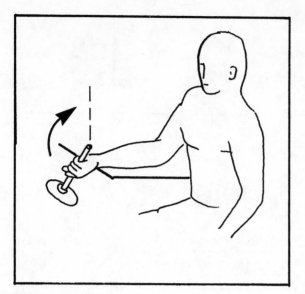

Figure 12-14

Forearm Supinations

Obtain a bar that is weighted on the end. Sit at a table and place your hand over the edge. With the palm turned up, rotate the bar until it points toward the ceiling (Fig. 12-14).

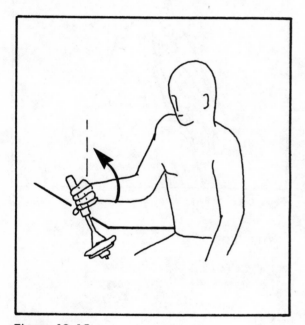

Figure 12-15

Forearm Pronation

Take the same position as in the exercise for forearm supination, but start with the palm turned down and rotate the bar toward the ceiling (Fig. 12-15).

NOTE: All the elbow exercises should be done twice daily. Do 4 sets of 10 repetitions. Once you have worked up to that number, gradually increase the weight to five pounds.

Edward J. Shahady

Wrist Injuries

Wrist injuries are common to all sports and usually consist of minor sprains, strains, or contusions, which readily heal with conservative treatment. However, **any wrist pain should be considered serious until proven otherwise**. Some painful chronic problems can develop that last a lifetime if a wrist injury receives improper treatment due to faulty diagnosis. **With wrist injuries, it is always best to err on the side of over-treatment**.

Several bones comprise the wrist, including the distal (lower) end of the forearm bones (radius and ulna) and a series of eight small bones (the carpals) that form the wrist joint. Figure 13-1 shows the wrist bones—the metacarpals, the radius, and the ulna.

The wrist can move in any one of six different ways: dorsiflexion (cocking the wrist) and palmarflexion, ulnar and radial deviation, and pronation and supination (rotating or twisting the hand so that the palm faces upward or downward) (Fig 13-2). Knowledge of these motions plays a major role in diagnosing wrist injuries.

Scaphoid/Navicular Fracture

Description

The scaphoid/navicular bone, located on the radial side of the wrist, accounts for 70 percent of wrist fractures (Fig. 13-3). A scaphoid fracture often results when an athlete falls directly on the open palm with the wrist dorsiflexed.

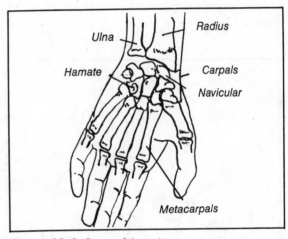

Figure 13-1. Bones of the wrist

Symptoms

- Pain on the radial side of the wrist
- Pain aggravated by strong gripping

Exam

- Palpate for tenderness over the **anatomical snuffbox** (Fig. 13-4).
- Grasp the injured wrist and firmly resist the athlete's attempts to pronate and supinate the wrist (Fig. 13-4). Pain will accompany the athlete's efforts if the navicular bone is broken.

Treatment

- If the circumstances of the injury and the physical exam indicate a scaphoid/navicular fracture, refer to a physician for X rays.

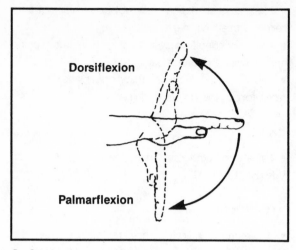

A. Cocking the wrist

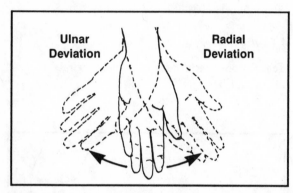

B. Ulnar and radial deviation

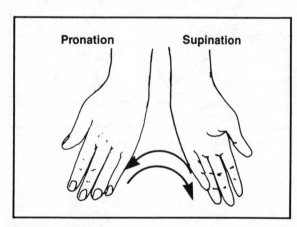

C. Wrist rotation

Figure 13-2. Wrist movements

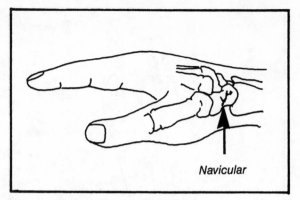

Figure 13-3. Scaphoid/navicular fracture

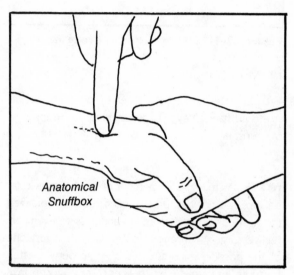

Figure 13-4. Location of the anatomical snuffbox

• Often a fracture may fail to show up on an X ray until two weeks after the injury. If the initial X ray is negative, but the physician suspects a fracture, the athlete is often placed in a short arm cast that encases both the forearm and the thumb until the wrist can be X-rayed again in two to three weeks.

Rehabilitation

• Athletes with broken wrists usually cannot return to competition until the fracture heals. Occasionally, however, a combination of casts—silicone for competition and plaster at all other times—will allow an athlete to compete, depending on the location of the break in the scaphoid and the requirements for the particular sport.

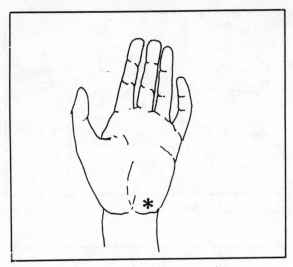

Figure 13-5. Location of pain with a hamate fracture

Prevention

Warn athletes about the danger of falling on an outstretched hand. Never underestimate the seriousness of a wrist injury.

NOTE: As many as 40 percent of scaphoid navicular fractures do not heal properly and require prolonged casting—up to 3 or 4 months—and possibly even corrective surgery. Chronic disabling arthritis is just one of the possible consequences of improperly treated fractures. If an athlete experiences chronic wrist pain in the anatomical snuffbox but has had a negative X ray, do not hesitate to suggest another examination by a physician.

Fracture of the Hamate

Description

The second most common wrist fracture involves the hook of the hamate. Such a fracture often results when a tennis player loses control of the racket while making a difficult shot or when a golfer misses a swing and slams the club into the ground.

Symptoms

• Pain over the ulnar side of the wrist and palm (Fig. 13-5).

• Normal wrist motions may not be painful, but pain recurs with athletic participation.
• Ordinary gripping may not induce pain, but gripping and swinging a club or a bat causes pain.
• Pain becomes so intense that performance deteriorates, forcing the athlete to quit.

Exam

• Palpate for tenderness over the palm on the ulnar side (Fig. 13-6).

Treatment

• If symptoms indicate a hamate fracture, refer the athlete to a physician for examination.
• Treatment can include a cast or surgery; the athlete should be able to return to activity in 6 weeks.

Prevention

Teach proper techniques for handling a racket, club, or bat.

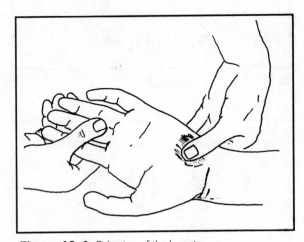

Figure 13-6. Palpation of the hamate

Tendinitis

Description

Wrist tendons are long, fibrous bands of tissue that connect muscles to bones. They either attach to the wrist bones or bypass the wrist and attach to the metacarpal or finger bones. Repeated, prolonged use or a sudden and substantial increase in use of these tendons can cause inflammation, pain, and limited movement. Tendinitis is most common in such sports as gymnastics, tennis, golf, and track (discus and shotput).

Symptoms

• Persistent pain, something like a toothache.
• Pain may have been present for "a while."
• Pain is dull and vague at rest but becomes severe with gripping.
• Grip becomes weak.
• Athlete may report a "squeaking" of the tendon or a feeling that a finger is "caught" when trying to straighten it out.

Exam

• Palpate for tenderness (Fig. 13-7).
• Check to see if the tendon actually feels thicker or has a knot in it at the point of tenderness.
• Grasp the injured wrist and firmly resist the athlete's attempts to move the wrist in several directions. Pain indicates tendinitis.

Treatment

• Splint the wrist (Fig. 13-8) and have the athlete take nonsteroidal anti-inflammatories.

Rehabilitation

• Tendinitis may require a slow return to participation punctuated by intermittent periods of splinting the wrist. Many athletes have difficulty decreasing their practice routine and consequently continue to experience discomfort for a long period of time.
• Athletes with recurring tendinitis should be referred to a physician.

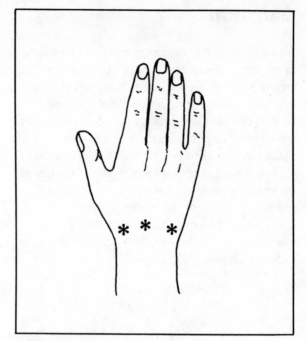

Figure 13-7. Location of tendinitis pain

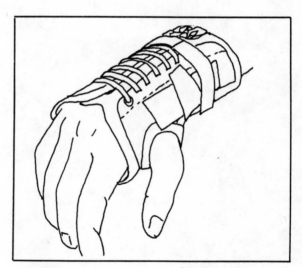

Figure 13-8. Wrist splint

Ganglion

A ganglion is a lump that can appear either on the top or bottom of the wrist (Fig. 13-9). The lump appears gradually and can grow to the size of a pea or a large marble. A ganglion feels soft and slightly movable. The lump can be painful, but usually its appearance causes more concern than actual pain.

Controversy surrounds treatment of ganglia. Many physicians feel that nothing needs to be done as long as the athlete is able to perform without pain. Some physicians advocate cortisone injections, and some advocate surgery. It is not unusual for ganglia to reappear after any type of treatment. They also can disappear without treatment.

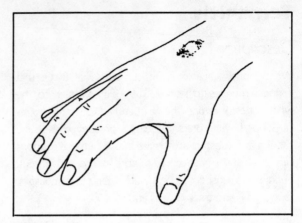

Figure 13-9. Ganglion

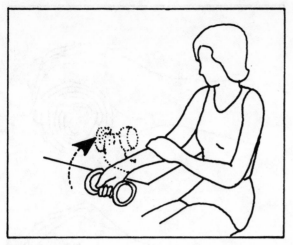
Figure 13-10

Wrist Exercises

Wrist Flexion

• Sit with the arm supported by a table and the wrist extended over the edge with the palm facing up. Slowly lift a weight and lower it back down (Fig. 13-10).

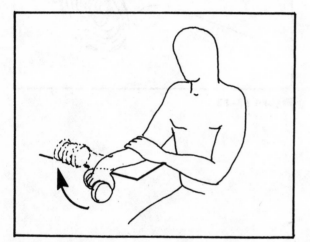
Figure 13-11

Wrist Extension

• Use the same position as in the wrist flexion exercise, but turn the palm toward the floor and extend the wrist, then lower the weight back to its original position (Fig. 13-11).

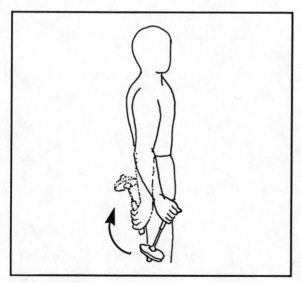
Figure 13-12

Ulnar Deviation

• Stand with the arm to the side and hold a bar with a weight on one end, pointed downward (Fig. 13-12). Lift the weight by palmarflexing the wrist and return slowly to original position.

Grip and Squeeze

• Hold a squeezable elastic bandage in the injured hand. Squeeze it tightly and then relax (Fig. 13-13).

NOTE: Wrist exercises should be done twice daily. Do 4 to 5 sets of 10 repetitions to help increase strength. Start with a two-pound weight and gradually add weight.

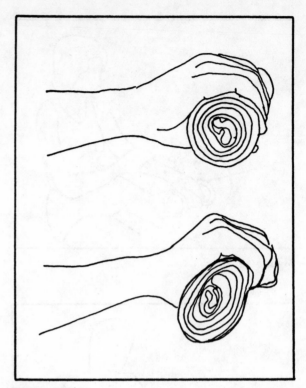

Figure 13-13

Edward J. Shahady

14

Hand/Finger Injuries

Hand injuries occur in most sports. Though most hand injuries consist of mild to moderate bruises or sprains, differentiating between the milder injuries and more serious injuries that can produce permanent disabilities or cosmetic defects (deformities) can be challenging, and for this reason no hand injury should be taken lightly.

Nineteen small bones (five metacarpals and fourteen phalanges) and a multitude of ligaments and tendons combine to form the hand (Fig. 14-1). The thumb has two phalanges, whereas the fingers have three phalanges each. These structures allow the hand to perform very complex functions.

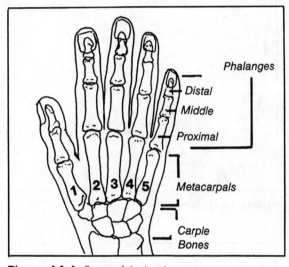

Figure 14-1. Bones of the hand

Hand Injuries

Metacarpal Fractures

(Broken Hand)

Description

Metacarpals can fracture in four possible locations: the neck, the shaft, the base, or the head (Fig. 14-2). These fractures produce pain and swelling or deformity. **The most frequently fractured metacarpal neck is the fifth**, an injury often referred to as a "boxer's fracture" because it results from a clenched fist striking a rigid object (Fig. 14-3). The initial X ray sometimes

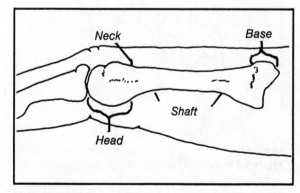

Figure 14-2. Fracture locations

79

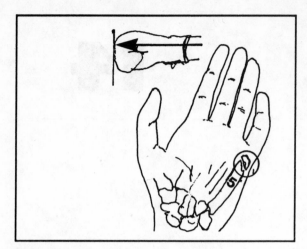

Figure 14-3. Boxer's fracture

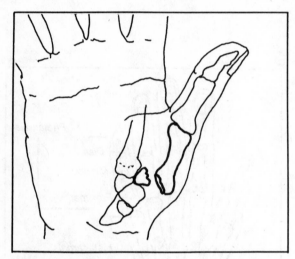

Figure 14-4. Bennett's fracture

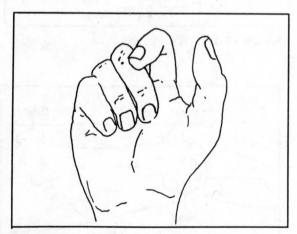

Figure 14-5. Fractured shaft of second metacarpal

misses fractures of the metacarpal base, so an athlete with persistent pain and swelling in that area may need more than one set of X rays. The thumb metacarpal is most commonly fractured at the base, an injury known as "Bennett's fracture," and is often associated with a dislocation (Fig. 14-4). Bennett's fracture, like boxer's fracture, is the result of striking an object with a closed fist and requires surgical treatment.

Symptoms

• **Metacarpal neck**—fractures of the fifth or second metacarpal produce a visible deformity. The broken bone points upward away from the palm, making a pronounced bump. Because the third and fourth metacarpals have better ligamentous support, a fracture of these bones does not produce a deformity.
• **Metacarpal shaft**—fractures of the shaft sometimes cause rotation of the fingers (Fig. 14-5).
• **Metacarpal base**—characterized by persistent pain and swelling over the base.

Exam

• To test for a shaft fracture, have the athlete make a fist. Examine the fingers for signs of rotation (see Fig. 14-5).
• Palpate each of the metacarpals for signs of a break (Fig. 14-6).

Treatment

• Ice and splint the finger until it can be X-rayed.
• Refer athletes with a suspected fracture to a physician.
• Many of these athletes may return to practice and participation after a short period of recovery if they wear a special cast recommended by the team physician.

Thumb Sprain

(Gamekeeper's Thumb)

Description

With this injury, the ligament that attaches to the proximal phalanx of the thumb and the thumb metacarpal (the ulnar collateral) is torn or partially torn (Fig. 14-7). It is particularly common in such sports as football, wrestling, and baseball.

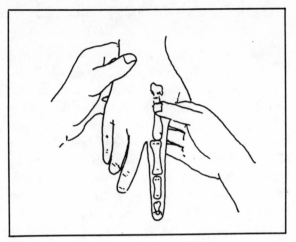

Figure 14-6. Palpation of the second metacarpal

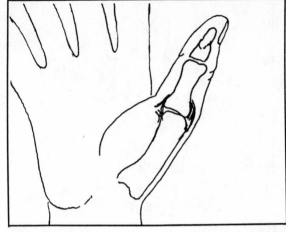

Figure 14-7. Tear in ulnar collateral ligament of the thumb

Symptoms

• The athlete experiences mild pain over the joint at rest and severe pain when the thumb is pulled away from the hand or when gripping.
• Swelling of the joint.

Exam

• Palpate the ulnar ligament for tenderness.
• Stretch the joint away from the hand and see if the movement causes pain (Fig. 14-8).
• Compare the injured with the uninjured thumb; check for swelling and instability.

Treatment

• Partial tears with no instability must be protected from further injury by taping the thumb to the hand (Fig 14-9A).
• If the athlete needs to use the thumb, use a figure-eight bandage, which will act as a restraint to prevent the thumb from stretching too far (Fig. 14-9B).
• Refer an athlete who experiences thumb instability or point tenderness over the bone to a physician.

Contusions to the Top of the Hand

An athlete may come to the trainer one or two weeks after an injury to complain of a lump forming over one of the metacarpals. Calcification (hardening) of old blood that has not been absorbed following the pri-

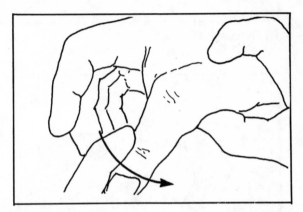

Figure 14-8. Testing the ulnar collateral ligament of the thumb for pain and stability

mary injury often causes this lump on the top of the hand. **A lump caused by calcification is usually painless and is not considered serious**. However, if the lump is painful and appears to be part of the metacarpal bone, it could indicate a healing fracture, and the athlete should see a physician.

Contusions to the Bottom of the Hand

Contusions to the bottom (or palm) of the hand can be quite disabling because the palm has very little room for swelling. Any injury that creates swelling requires ice, protection, and rest until the swelling dissipates. If an athlete complains of numbness or tingling of the fingers or inability to move the fingers, have the athlete see a physician.

Phalanges (Finger) Injuries

The three bones (phalanges) that comprise each finger are the most commonly fractured bones in the body. The **proximal phalanx** is fractured more than the **middle** or the **distal phalanx** (Fig. 14-10). Many of the tendons attached to these finger bones can tear with or without a fracture, and the three joints—the **DIP** (distal interphalangeal), **PIP** (proximal interphalangeal), and **MCP** (metacarpal phalangeal)—can also suffer injury. Keep a few basics in mind when caring for finger injuries:

• **How the injury occurred**. Was the finger pushed too far backward or forward?
• **Location of pain**.
• **Presence or absence of instability**. Stable joints don't allow movement beyond their normal range. But when a muscle or tendon tears, there is increased movement.

Drop (Mallet) Finger

(Extensor Tendon Tear)

Description

Mallet finger occurs when impact forces the fingertip too far downward (flexion), often as the result of a hard thrown ball striking the fingertip (Fig. 14-11). This injury is common in such sports as football (receivers), baseball (catchers), and basketball.

Symptoms

• Immediate pain in fingertip.
• Athlete usually stops and seeks immediate attention but sometimes will not see the trainer until "drop finger" appears.
• Athlete is unable to extend (straighten) the fingertip.
• The DIP joint is swollen.

Exam

• Palpate for tenderness over the dorsum (top) of the finger at the DIP joint.
• Examine the DIP joint for swelling or deformity. When first injured, the finger may not look "dropped" because of the swelling. The characteristic deformity appears one to two weeks later if the injury is not properly treated.

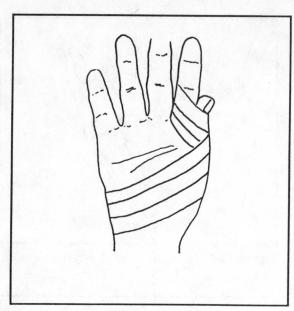

A. Thumb taped for non-ball handler

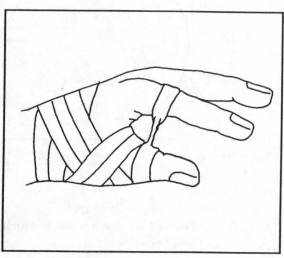

B. Thumb taped for ball handler

Figure 14-9. Taping for thumb sprain

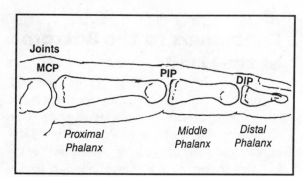

Figure 14-10. Phalanges and phalangeal joints

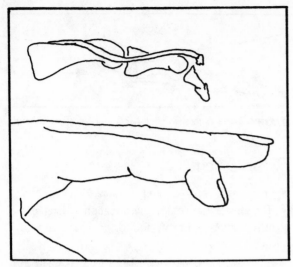

Figure 14-11. Tearaway of the extensor tendon from the base of the distal phalanx, with characteristic mallet finger deformity

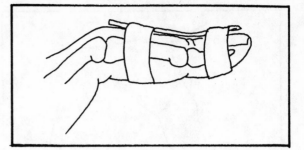

Figure 14-12. Splint for mallet finger

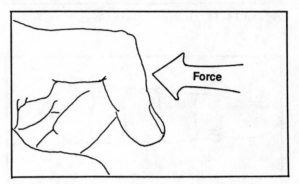

Figure 14-13. Hyperflexion of the finger

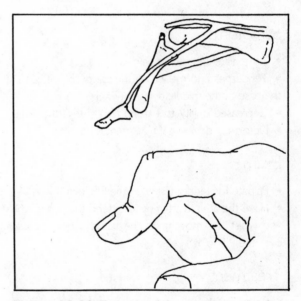

Figure 14-14. Tearaway of the extensor tendon from the base of the middle phalanx, with characteristic boutonniere deformity

Treatment

• Splint the DIP joint in an extended position for 6 weeks full time and for 6 more weeks at night (Fig. 14-12). The PIP joint should not be involved in the splinting but should remain free.

• Refer an athlete with extreme tenderness or marked deformity of the fingertip to a physician for evaluation. If the diagnosis is delayed, the finger should be splinted for 6 to 10 weeks after the injury; however, delaying treatment can adversely affect the finger's recovery.

• In most cases, athletes can participate if they wear a splint.

Boutonniere (Buttonhole) Finger

(Sprained Finger)

Description

Boutonniere finger, another of the so-called sprained fingers, occurs when a sudden impact causes the finger to hyperflex (Fig. 14-13), rupturing the extensor ligament over the PIP joint (Fig. 14-14). This joint, or knuckle, slips between two parts of the extensor tendon like a button through a buttonhole.

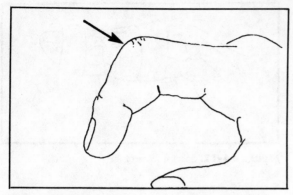

Figure 14-15. Location of pain with boutonniere injury

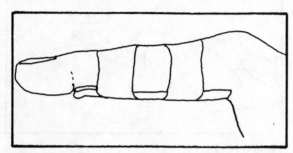

Figure 14-16. Splint for boutonniere finger

Symptoms

- Immediate and severe pain.
- Tenderness, normally over the top of the PIP joint at the base of the middle phalanx (Fig. 14-15).
- Decreased ability to extend (straighten) the finger.
- Deformity develops if treatment is delayed.

Exam

- Palpate for tenderness over the PIP joint.
- Have the athlete attempt to extend the finger while you resist the movement; the result should be pain over the PIP joint.

Treatment

- Refer an athlete with boutonniere finger symptoms to a physician.
- Splint the PIP joint, fully extended, for 1 week and then reevaluate. If tenderness and difficulty extending the finger persist, continue the splint for 3 more weeks. The splint should not limit the movement of the MCP or DIP joints (Fig. 14-16).

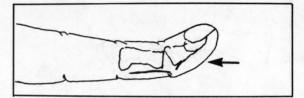

Figure 14-17. Jersey finger—tearaway of flexor tendon

Rehabilitation

- Encourage flexion of the DIP joint.
- The athlete can resume participation as long as the joint is splinted and protected for an additional 6 to 8 weeks.
- A misdiagnosed injury can still be treated as late as 8 to 10 weeks afterward by splinting the finger.

Jersey Finger
(Deep Flexor Tendon Tear)

Description

Jersey finger involves the flexor tendon that attaches to the distal phalanx. This tendon can tear when the finger catches in a jersey or belt loop, forcing the finger to extend (bend backward) beyond its normal range (Fig. 14-17). Ring fingers tend to suffer torn flexor tendons more than other fingers.

Symptoms

- Sudden pain in the fingertip while grabbing a jersey

Exam

- Examine the underneath (volar) part of the fingertip for tenderness and swelling.
- The most distinct characteristic of a jersey finger is the athlete's inability to flex the DIP joint (Fig. 14-18). Tenderness and swelling alone will not prevent finger flexion.

Treatment

- The athlete may wait 24 to 48 hours before seeing a physician if the diagnosis is in doubt. However, correcting a tear requires surgery and waiting more than 5 days can jeopardize the success of surgery.

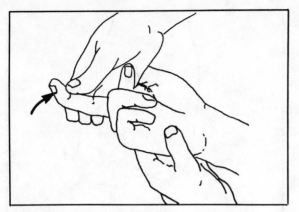

Figure 14-18. Testing for flexor of the DIP joint

Stowed Finger

(Volar Plate Fracture)

Description

Stowed fingers occur when a finger gets pushed too far backward (hyperextended) at the PIP joint (Fig. 14-19). Hyperextension often leads to dislocation of a finger joint. Other athletes with a swollen or tender PIP joint may have a small volar plate fracture.

Symptoms

• PIP joint begins swelling within a few hours.
• Because the discomfort increases in severity over time, athletes often delay bringing the injury to a trainer's or coach's attention until after a game or practice, or even until the next day.

Exam

• Check for weakness and tenderness of the PIP joint at the base of the middle phalanx when the finger is extended (Fig. 14-20).

Treatment

• Any athlete with a swollen PIP joint should have the finger X-rayed immediately. An improperly treated volar plate fracture will cause a deformity that can only be corrected through surgery.
• The injured finger should be splinted with the PIP joint flexed to approximately 20 to 30 degrees for 3 or 4 weeks. Such a splint is usually applied to the top side of the finger (Fig. 14-21).

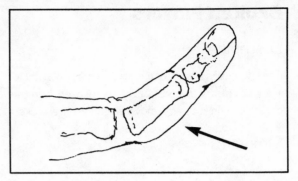

Figure 14-19. Hyperextended finger

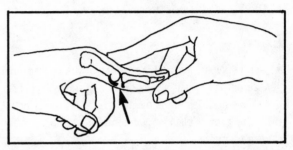

Figure 14-20. Stress test shows an increase in extension of PIP joint with volar plate injury

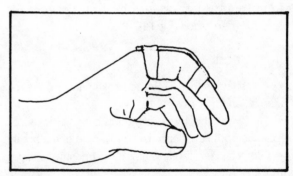

Figure 14-21. Splinting of the PIP joint for volar plate hyperextension injuries

• If the finger is adequately protected, the athlete may continue participation.
• After 3 to 4 weeks in a splint, the finger should be "buddy taped" for another 2 to 3 weeks as the athlete returns to full participation.

Broken Fingers

Description

Fingers usually break as the result of a direct hit or a fall. Contrary to popular belief, broken bones—particularly fingers—can move when they are broken.

Symptoms

- Immediate pain.
- The finger hurts with or without movement.
- Swelling.
- The finger may look "twisted."

Exam

- Gently palpate each of the bones of the injured finger. Using one finger, slowly feel along the injured finger above and below the painful area and then directly over the area itself. Pinpoint tenderness usually indicates a fracture.
- Because of tendon attachments and muscle forces, fractures of the middle and proximal phalanx may cause visible and palpable deformities. Ask the athlete to make a half-fist with each hand and compare nail lines for malrotation (Fig. 14-22).

Treatment

- An athlete with a suspected broken finger must see a physician for X rays.
- The finger should be splinted in either a flexed or extended position, depending on location of the break.
- Buddy taping is rarely sufficient treatment for a finger fracture.

Sprained Fingers

(Collateral Ligament Injuries)

Description

The DIP and PIP joints both have a ligament on either side of the joint (Fig. 14-23). One of these, the radial collateral ligament, is the most commonly sprained or torn finger ligament. The less commonly injured ligament is the ulnar collateral ligament. These sprains usually result when a ball or other dull object strikes the finger and bends it sideways.

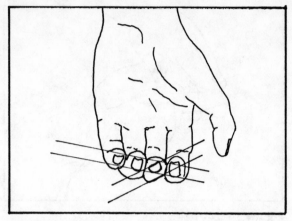

Figure 14-22. The nail line of the second finger is not parallel to the others, usually indicating a fractured middle or proximal phalanx

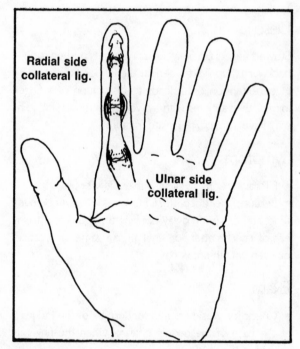

Radial side collateral lig.

Ulnar side collateral lig.

Figure 14-23. Collateral ligaments

Symptoms

- Severe pain and swelling over the collateral ligament at the PIP joint

Exam

- Palpate the sides of the PIP and DIP joints for tenderness. Pain is located directly over the side of the joint rather than below the joint (volar plate fracture) or above the joint (boutonniere injury).

• Perform the **collateral ligament stress test** by grasping the end of the injured finger and stressing the joint to see if there is excess movement (Fig. 14-24). This test reveals pain or weakness in the ligaments that is not noticeable with normal extension or flexion.

Treatment

• If there is no instability in the joint, splint the finger in a flexed position (20 to 30 degrees) until the pain subsides. The athlete may continue participation but should protect the finger by buddy taping it to an adjacent finger.
• If instability exists, refer the athlete to a physician.

Dislocations

Dislocations are common and often can be reduced (put back in place) on the field by the coach or trainer. However, you should be aware of certain features of dislocations before you attempt to relocate one:
• Gentle, steady traction (pulling) is usually sufficient to reduce the dislocation. **Never try to force a stubborn dislocation back into place**.
• Because many dislocations are associated with a fracture, a follow-up X ray is usually advisable.
• The finger should be protected by splinting for 3 weeks and buddy taping for another 3 weeks after the dislocation has been reduced.
• Volar plate injuries can be associated with dislocations at the PIP joint, so finger should be splinted as shown in Figure 14-21.

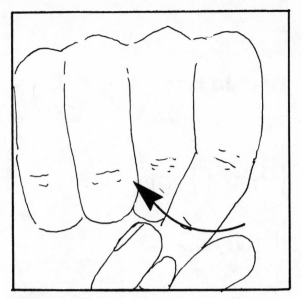

Figure 14-24. Stress test for collateral ligament weakness

Subungual Hematoma

(Blood under Fingernail)

Fingertips are commonly exposed to sources of trauma that cause bleeding underneath the fingernail. This condition is usually very painful because of the pressure created by blood pressing against the nail. Making a hole in the nail with a sharp disposable needle or a hot paper clip relieves the pain and also prevents the nail from falling off in the future. This technique can be learned from the team physician but **should not be tried without some prior experience or supervision**.

Donald Ives

15

Hip/Thigh Injuries

Hip Injuries

The most common hip injuries are muscle and tendon strains. The seriousness of each strain varies, depending on the amount of torn muscle fiber. Compared with injuries to other parts of the body, hip injuries are relatively uncommon in high school athletics and usually result from overuse (82 percent) rather than from trauma (18 percent). Running (which alone accounts for 61 percent of hip injuries), fitness training, and racket and collision sports carry the highest risk of hip injury. Hip injuries are frustrating because they tend to be persistent and do not respond to initial treatment.

The hip joint is a close-fitting, ball-in-socket joint composed of the **acetabulum** (the socket), on the outer wall of the pelvis, and the head of the **femur** (the ball). Four large muscle groups that originate above the hip, pass over the joint to form the muscles of the thigh, and attach to the thighbone (femur) or shinbone (tibia) provide mobility (Fig. 15-1). Depending on their location, these muscles permit motion in four directions—forward (flexion), backward (extension), to the outside (abduction), and to the inside (adduction) (Fig. 15-2). Hip injuries usually take the form of damage to one or more of these muscle groups.

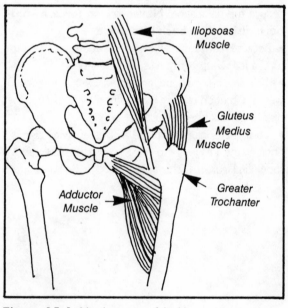

Figure 15-1. Muscle groups of the hip

Groin (Adductor) Strain
(Pulled Groin Muscle)

Description

Groin strains are caused by an acute or abrupt change of direction or by twisting the thigh while the legs are

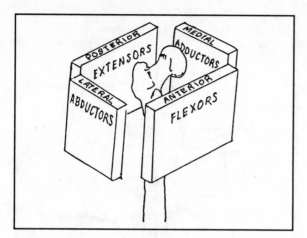

Figure 15-2. Hip muscles by quadrant

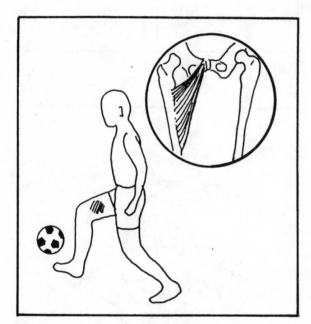

Figure 15-3. Adductor (groin) strain

spread wide apart. They often occur on muddy fields during running and kicking sports (Fig. 15-3).

Symptoms

• The athlete walks with a limp and complains of a soreness in the groin that radiates to the inner part of the thigh.

Exam

• Test the adductor muscle for strength by applying resistance as the athlete crosses his or her legs (Fig. 15-4). In the presence of a groin strain, this movement will elicit pain.

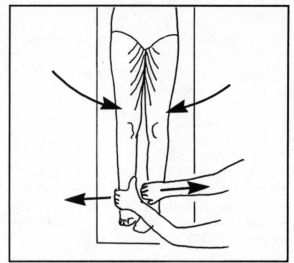

Figure 15-4. Adductor muscle test

Treatment and Prevention

• See "Treatment for Muscle Strains" below.

Flexor (Iliopsoas) Strain
(Deep Groin Strain)

Description

Flexor strains are caused by a vigorous attempt to bring the leg forward while the thigh is fixed or forced into extension (Fig. 15-5).

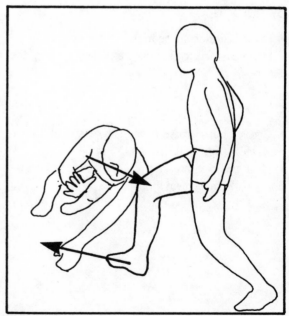

Figure 15-5. Injury to iliopsoas

Symptoms

• The athlete complains of deep groin tenderness and pain that radiates into the lower abdomen.
• The athlete may hold the thigh in a flexed, crossed, and externally rotated position.

Exam

• Check to see if attempts to move the hip backward or forward or to rotate the leg cause severe pain.
• Check for pain when the hip is flexed against the examiner's resistance (Fig. 15-6).
• Palpate for tenderness in the area of the **lesser trochanter** (Fig. 15-7).

Treatment and Prevention

• See "Treatment for Muscle Strains" below.

Abductor (Gluteus Medius) Strain

(Hip Strain)

Description

This injury usually results from overuse of the gluteus medius. Its symptoms are easily confused with those of trochanteric bursitis.

Symptoms

• Pain radiates down the thigh to the knee.
• Hip movement causes pain, especially crossing the legs.

Exam

• Check for an increase in pain with resisted abduction movement (Fig. 15-8).
• Move the joint through the full range of passive motion. Passive movement should cause no pain.

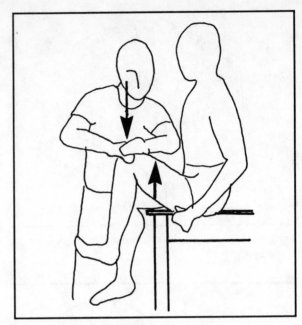

Figure 15-6. Test for iliopsoas strain

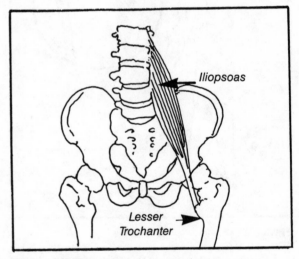

Figure 15-7. Location of lesser trochanter

Treatment and Prevention

• See "Treatment for Muscle Strains" below.

Treatment for Muscle Strains

• Treat the acute symptoms. Reduce pain, swelling, and inflammation by elevating the leg and applying ice immediately. Apply a compressive wrap (Ace bandage). The athlete should rest to allow the injury time to heal.

Do not allow the athlete to practice or play injured as this increases the risk of reinjury and serious damage.

• Once the acute symptoms subside, the goal for trainer and athlete should be to restore normal motion, minimize scar formation, and retard muscular atrophy. Apply alternate cold and hot packs (10 minutes each), to be followed with gentle, pain-free exercises covering the joint's entire range of motion, performed in a whirlpool. In cases of persistent or particularly severe pain, an X ray may be necessary in order to rule out the possibility of a fracture.

• The next goal is the recovery of normal strength and flexibility. The athlete begins gentle stretching and isometric (tightening the muscle without moving the leg) exercises, followed gradually by exercises with weights. **Keep in mind that rushing the healing process may result in a more severe strain or permanent damage**. The athlete should stop an exercise immediately if it causes any pain.

• The athlete may return to competition upon regaining 90 percent strength compared to the uninjured side, complete flexibility, and full range of motion without pain.

Prevention of Muscle Strains

Many muscle strains can be avoided by paying careful attention to proper warm-up and thorough stretching exercises. Coaches should delay the beginning of "crossover drills" for the first few weeks of practice until the athletes are in shape.

Trochanteric Bursitis

(Chronic Hip Pain)

Description

The **trochanteric bursa** separates the bony greater trochanter of the femur and the overlying muscle. It provides lubrication and padding during motion. Trochanteric bursitis occurs when the bursa becomes irritated or inflamed as the result of a direct blow, an infection, or overuse. Runners often develop bursitis from running on banked surfaces or due to abnormal running mechanics (e.g., feet crossing the midline) or structural flaws in the body (e.g., a discrepancy in leg lengths). The condition is more common in female athletes because a broader pelvis increases the mechanical stress placed on hip structures.

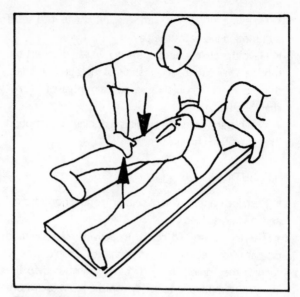

Figure 15-8. Abduction test for gluteus medius

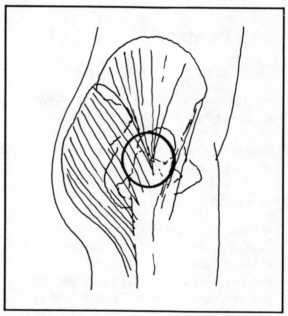

Figure 15-9. Pain area for trochanteric bursitis

Symptoms

• The athlete complains of pain that radiates down the thigh to the knee.

• Hip movement, specifically crossing the legs, is painful.

Exam

• Palpate (feel) for tenderness over the greater trochanter (Fig. 15-9).

- Have the athlete cross the leg and rotate it to see if that motion increases the pain.
- Have the athlete abduct the hip while you resist the motion. Unlike tendinitis or strain of the gluteus medius, the movement should cause no pain in cases of trochanteric bursitis.
- Audible and palpable crepitus (grinding) with motion may indicate a chronic condition.

Treatment

- Rest, local application of heat or ice, and nonsteroidal anti-inflammatories.
- The athlete should return to activity gradually, and only after correcting any biomechanical problems (e.g., running mechanics) that may have contributed to the injury. It is important to redevelop the hip musculature with hip-strengthening exercises. It may be necessary to refer the athlete to a physician for a full evaluation.

Hip Pointer

Description

A hip pointer essentially is a bruise or muscle tear over the pelvic bone (iliac crest). It results from a direct blow to the unprotected prominence of the pelvic bone. It is most likely to occur in contact sports such as football (Fig. 15-10).

Symptoms

- Athleté may experience immediate, momentarily incapacitating pain in the region of the iliac crest.
- The pain should diminish with rest.
- Alternatively, in the heat of a game the athlete may feel no immediate pain but, in the ensuing 24 hours, may experience substantial edema, pain, and discoloration.

Exam

- Palpate for tenderness directly over the iliac crest (Fig. 15-11).
- Be aware of general pain in the area. Because the iliac crest is the site of insertion for hip abductor and

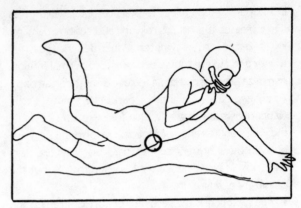

Figure 15-10. Sustaining a hip pointer

flexor muscles as well as abdominal muscles, motion involving any of these groups (including bending or twisting the trunk) is painful. The athlete often has difficulty standing upright and walking normally because of pain and muscle spasm.

Treatment

- Apply ice and elastic compresses and restrict activity until symptoms subside. Occasionally an athlete will require crutches for a few days.
- The athlete should return to activity slowly after the pain subsides, usually within a period of 2 to 3 weeks.

Prevention

Routine use of properly fitting hip pads should be effective in preventing most hip pointers.

Femoral Neck Stress Fractures

Description

A stress fracture occurs most often in running sports. Although this is an uncommon injury, the consequences can be serious. If the fracture disrupts the flow of blood to the femoral head, the athlete can be permanently disabled. Thus, a thorough evaluation is essential.

Symptoms

- The athlete may experience vague, deep tenderness on the anterior (front) side of the hip during activity and may walk with a limp.

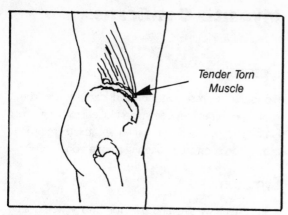

Figure 15-11. Location of pain with a hip pointer

• As weeks go by, the pain may begin earlier during activity and persist longer, but it usually disappears after 48 hours of rest.

Exam

• Check for a decreased ability to move the hip in all directions without causing pain.
• Perform tests for muscle strength (flexion, extension, abduction, and adduction) to see if they reveal weakness and cause pain.

Treatment

• Be suspicious of pain that has no apparent cause. It is very important to diagnose this injury correctly.
• Refer the athlete to a physician for X rays. Give the physician a complete account of the athlete's symptoms.
• The athlete must rest a fractured hip for 3 to 5 weeks, followed by a gradual return to full activity.

Thigh Injuries

The thigh consists of a single bone, the thighbone (femur), which is surrounded and protected by heavy muscle. These muscles originate in the pelvis and insert on the femur or proximal tibia. As a result, most injuries to the thigh are muscular injuries. Treatment is similar to the treatment for other muscle injuries (see "Treatment for Muscle Strains" above).

Quadriceps Contusion

(Charley Horse)

Description

The quadriceps muscle pulls the knee into extension (see Chapter 16, "Knee Injuries"). A charley horse essentially is a bruised quadriceps muscle. It results from a direct blow to the anterior thigh (Fig. 15-12).

Symptoms

• Typically, the athlete feels some initial discomfort in the area of the blow but often continues playing.
• The athlete later develops a limp, pain, swelling, and discoloration (Fig. 15-13).
• Alternatively, the athlete may be disabled immediately with severe pain in the thigh.

Exam

• Examine the athlete for three grades of quadriceps contusions (Fig. 15-14):
Grade 1. Mild contusion, tender over quadriceps. Athlete has no trouble walking, can flex (bend) the knee to 90 degrees or more, and can do knee bends easily.
Grade 2. Moderate contusion, tenderness and swelling over the quadriceps. Athlete walks with a limp but can do partial knee bends and is able to flex the knee to 60 degrees.
Grade 3. Severe contusion, marked swelling and tenderness; examiner is unable to feel the muscle contour. Athlete is unable to walk without help and can bend the knee only to 45 degrees or less.

Treatment

• Do not be complacent when treating quadriceps contusions. Grade 1 injuries heal in 3 to 5 days, but Grade 2 contusions take 2 to 3 weeks and a Grade 3 injury may sideline the athlete for the season. Bed rest, ice, elevation of the leg, and compression are the main elements of treatment. Myositis ossificans (see below) occurs in 70 percent of athletes with Grade 3 injuries. Physician referral and extensive rehabilitation are usually necessary with Grade 2 and 3 injuries.

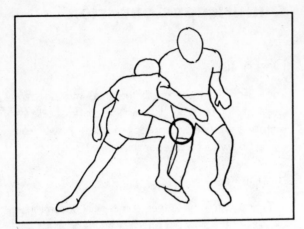

Figure 15-12. Thigh contusion

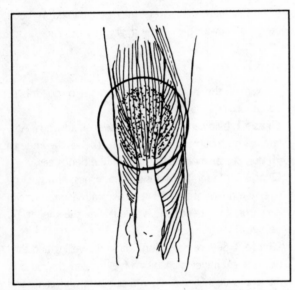

Figure 15-13. Thigh contusion (interior view)

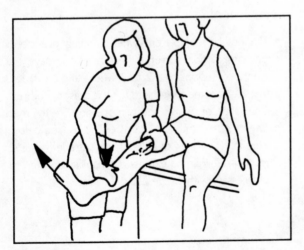

Figure 15-14. Quadriceps muscle test

Myositis Ossificans

(Bone in Muscle)

Description

Blood that is present in the quadriceps muscle from a contusion sometimes becomes calcified, forming a hard lump. This usually occurs when an athlete returns to activity too soon after suffering a contusion.

Symptoms

• Persistent swelling and pain for 2 to 4 weeks after the initial injury.

Exam

• Palpate for a tender, warm, hard mass over the thigh. There may also be swelling and limitation of knee movement.

Treatment

• Continued rest and treatment for recurrent contusion should cure this condition. Physician referral is indicated, but this is not a surgical problem; ask for another opinion if the physician suggests surgery.

Pulled Hamstring

(Hamstring Strain)

Description

A pulled hamstring commonly occurs in sports that involve sprinting. Basically, this injury is a tear in the muscle fibers. Hamstrings tear due to extreme stretching at the beginning of a sprint when the hip is flexed and the knee extended. The risk of a pulled hamstring increases when the athlete has not warmed up properly and tries a hurdle or a "jack-rabbit" start (Fig. 15-15).

Symptoms

• Pain in the posterior thigh while running, which causes a limp.

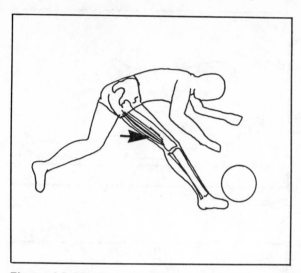

Figure 15-15. Hamstring tear

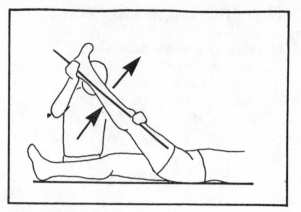

Figure 15-16. Straight leg raising test

Exam

• Palpate for tenderness. In a **first-degree strain**, the muscle tear causes little swelling and no visible defect. Pain increases with movements that stretch the hamstring, for example, the straight leg raising test (Fig. 15-16).

• A **second-degree strain** involves a partial disruption of the muscle. Muscle spasm causes the athlete to hold the knee in a flexed position. There is also some discoloration.

• A **third-degree strain** causes severe pain, swelling, and disability, and there may be an immediate palpable defect apparent in the muscle (Fig. 15-17).

Treatment

• Apply ice and elevate the leg immediately.

• Later, wrap the leg in a compressive bandage. These measures reduce swelling, pain, and edema. In severe cases the athlete may need to use crutches in order to allow the muscle to rest. For second- and third-degree strains, physician evaluation may be necessary.

• As pain, swelling, and disability diminish, the athlete may begin slow, steady stretching exercises to reestablish flexibility and full range of motion.

• Upon regaining full motion, the athlete may begin exercises to redevelop power and endurance in the hamstrings.

• If the athlete is overzealous in his or her attempt to return to competition, the stronger, uninjured quadriceps can overpower the hamstrings, predisposing the

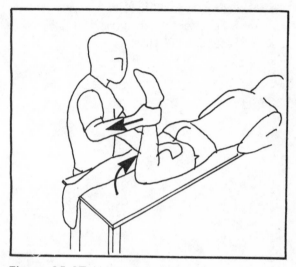

Figure 15-17. Hamstring muscle test

athlete to a recurrent strain syndrome. Complete healing sometimes takes 6 to 9 months.

• Extra warm-up and stretching exercises are a critical part of effective treatment.

Hip and Thigh Exercises

Hip Flexion (Iliopsoas Muscle)
• Lie on your back with one leg straight and the other knee bent. Bend the knee into the chest slowly (Fig. 15-18). Hold for 5 seconds and repeat 20 times. Repeat with the other leg.

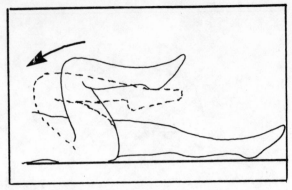

Figure 15-18

• Sit on a chair with feet flat on floor. Add a weight to the ankle of the affected leg (1 to 5 pounds). Slowly raise the knee toward the chest (Fig. 15-19). Hold for 5 seconds and repeat 20 times.

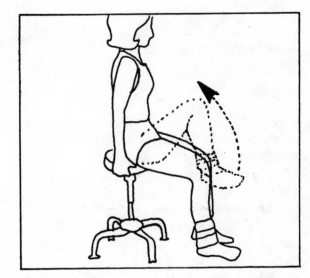

Figure 15-19

Hip Extension (Gluteus Maximus)
• Lie on your stomach. Place a weight (1 to 5 pounds) on one leg. Raise the leg above the hip slowly, keeping the knee straight (Fig. 15-20). Hold for 5 seconds and repeat 20 times. Repeat with other leg.

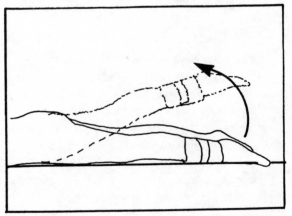

Figure 15-20

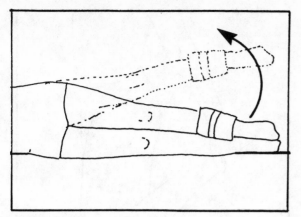

Figure 15-21

Outward Leg Raise (Gluteus Medius)

• Lie on your side with both legs straight and lift the outer leg up (Fig. 15-21). (This can be done with a weight on the ankle.) Hold each repetition for 5 seconds and repeat 20 times.

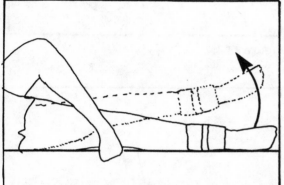
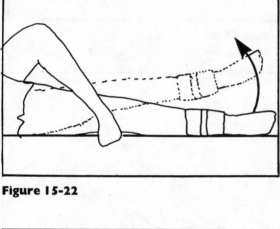

Figure 15-22

Inward Leg Raise (Adductor Muscle)

• Lie on your side with top leg bent over lower leg (Fig. 15-22). Lift the bottom leg upward. (A weight can be used.) Hold for 5 seconds and repeat 20 times.

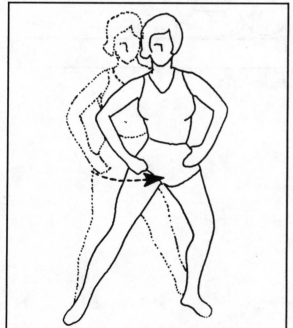

Figure 15-23

Adductor Stretch

• Stand straight with hands on hips. Lean to one side, keeping one leg straight and bending the other knee (Fig. 15-23). Hold for 5 seconds and repeat 10 times.

Stretching the Front of the Thigh (Quadriceps)

• Standing upright, grasp one foot and pull it toward the buttocks (Fig. 15-24). Hold for 5 seconds and repeat 30 times.

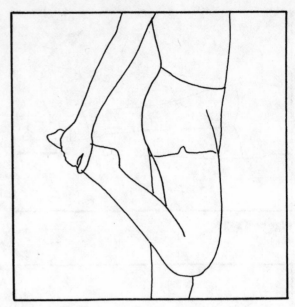

Figure 15-24

Stretching the Back of the Thigh (Hamstrings)

• While lying on your back, grasp one thigh and pull the leg toward your chest (Fig. 15-25). Keep your hips flat and the other leg straight. Hold for 5 seconds and repeat 10 times.

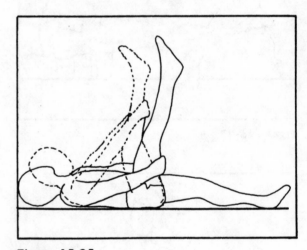

Figure 15-25

Mary G. Broos
Gregory H. Tuttle

16

Knee Injuries

Knee injuries plague athletes in practically every sport, accounting for 20 to 30 percent of all injuries. Knee injuries can be acute, resulting from contact such as a direct blow, or chronic, resulting from overuse of certain ligaments or tendons. Contact sports like football tend to produce torn ligaments, whereas sports that involve prolonged running, such as track and cross country, produce overuse injuries.

The knee consists of four bones (Fig. 16-1): the **femur** (thighbone), the **tibia** (shinbone), the **fibula** (a small, nonweightbearing bone), and the **patella** (kneecap). Knee joints work like hinges, allowing the lower leg to flex (bend), extend (straighten), and rotate, but they achieve mobility at the cost of stability. There-

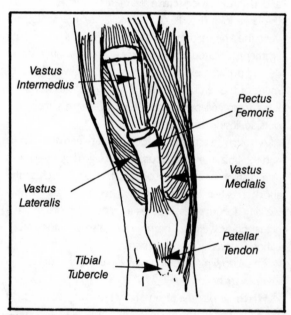

Figure 16-2. Four quadriceps muscles

fore knees depend on various muscles and ligaments for support. The **quadriceps** muscle, the large muscle in front of the thighbone, inserts into the top of the shinbone and extends the lower leg. The **hamstring** muscle, located behind the thighbone, inserts into the back of the shinbone and flexes the lower leg. Figure 16-2 shows the patella surrounded by the four quadriceps muscles as well as the **patellar tendon** and the **tibial tubercle**.

Four major ligaments—the **medial** (inside) and **lateral** (outside) **collateral** ligaments, and the **anterior**

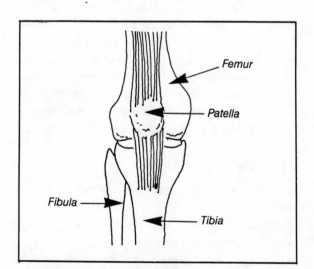

Figure 16-1. Four bones of the knee

99

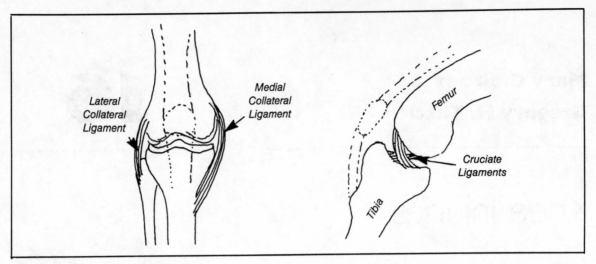

Figure 16-3. Ligaments of the knee

and **posterior cruciate** ligaments—further stabilize the knee joint (Fig. 16-3). The collateral ligaments prevent the knee from moving side to side. The cruciate ligaments, located inside the knee, provide inner stability and prevent excessive forward or backward movement of the femur and tibia. These ligaments keep the knee from collapsing when it receives stress from the outside, inside, back, or front.

A tough, elastic tissue located between the femur and the tibia, the **meniscus**, or cartilage (Fig. 16-4), acts as a cushion or shock absorber, absorbing much of the shock created by each step a person takes. Simple walking, for instance, creates a force three times one's actual body weight. The meniscus also provides lubrication for easy joint movement.

The following criteria deserve particular emphasis in knee examinations:

• **History**. Ask the athlete how the injury occurred, if the foot was planted firmly, if there was an accompanying pop or snap. If the injury resulted from a blow, determine the point of contact. Ask the athlete to show you where the knee hurts most and find out if either knee has been injured previously. Ask also if there has been a sudden increase in training time, a change of running surface, or a change in footwear.

• **Observation**. Always compare the injured knee with the uninjured one. Look for signs of physical deformity such as swelling or discoloration. Notice if the athlete walks with a limp or if there is an obvious loss of range of motion in the knee joint.

• **Palpation**. Feel the uninjured knee and then the injured one. It may be possible to feel fluid or defects in the tissue or bony structure of the knee. An injured knee may feel hot to the touch. Press the knee over the ligaments and cartilage to see if there is an area of mild to extreme pain.

Acute Knee Injuries

Anterior Cruciate Ligament Tear

Description

The anterior cruciate ligament (ACL) is located in the middle of the knee joint and prevents the lower leg from extending too far forward. A direct blow to the front of the knee that causes the lower leg to hyperextend often creates an ACL tear (Fig. 16-5). Rapid deceleration (slowing down) can also cause an ACL tear, as can cutting quickly or rotating the knee. ACL tears can be difficult to diagnose initially because some athletes may exhibit chronic (rather than acute) symptoms, such as the leg periodically giving out.

Symptoms

• The athlete hears a pop or feels something snap in the knee.
• The knee feels like it is going out of joint.
• There is immediate pain.
• The knee joint develops significant swelling immediately.

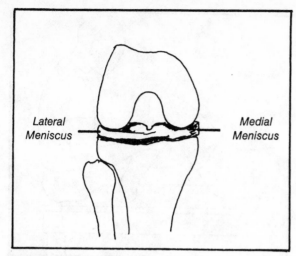

Figure 16-4. Knee cartilage

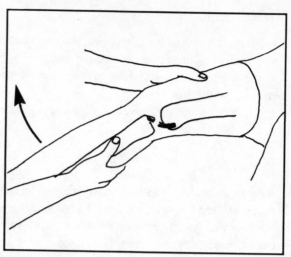

Figure 16-6. Lachman test

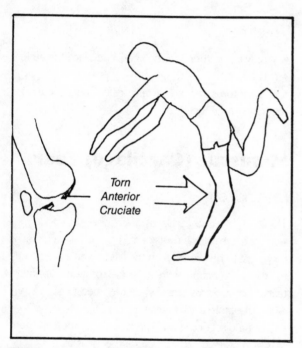

Figure 16-5. Hyperextended knee

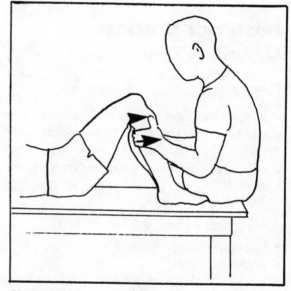

Figure 16-7. Anterior drawer test

Exam

• **The Lachman test**. With the athlete lying face up on a table, flex the injured knee to approximately 20 degrees. Check to be sure the athlete's hamstring muscles are relaxed. With one hand on the femur (thighbone) just above the knee to stabilize it, place the other hand on the tibia (shin) just below the knee and pull the tibia forward (Fig. 16-6). If the ligament is intact, the tibia comes to a firm stop. If the ligament is torn, the tibia continues forward sluggishly, as if attached to a rubber band. Significant swelling or pain that causes hamstring tightness may produce a negative exam result despite the presence of a torn ligament.

• **The anterior drawer test** is similar to the Lachman test. With the athlete reclining and both knees flexed to 90 degrees, stabilize the athlete's foot and pull the tibia forward with both hands, again checking for a firm stop (Fig. 16-7). This test is not as reliable as the Lachman test.

Treatment

• Elevate the injured knee, apply ice, and use a knee immobilizer to prevent the knee from bending.
• The athlete should use crutches to keep from putting weight on the injured knee.
• If symptoms indicate an ACL tear, refer the athlete to a physician.

Prevention

Athletes should follow a strengthening program for the quadriceps and hamstring muscles. The hamstrings are normally only half as strong as the quads. A program that increases hamstring strength to three-fourths or four-fifths that of the quads can help decrease knee injuries.

Posterior Cruciate Ligament Tear

Description

Posterior cruciate ligament tears are rare. They usually result from a direct blow to the front of the knee while the knee is bent and the foot planted. This injury is actually more common in automobile accidents than athletics.

Symptoms

• Possible swelling.
• The leg feels "loose."
• If pain is present, it is usually located behind the knee.

Exam

• **The posterior drawer test**. Have the athlete lie on a table with the knee bent to 90 degrees and the foot planted. Push the tibia backward toward the athlete (Fig. 16-8). In a positive test, the bone of the injured leg moves back further than the uninjured leg bone.
• **Knee bump test**. The athlete should be seated with both knees bent to 90 degrees and both feet planted. Look at both knees from the side at the point of the tibial tubercle and compare the knee bumps. With a posterior cruciate tear, the tibial tubercle will be less prominent on the injured side.

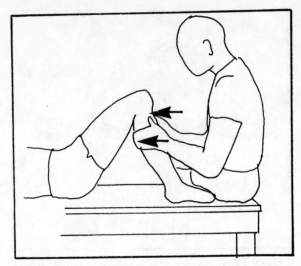

Figure 16-8. Posterior drawer test

Treatment

• Apply ice, immobilize the knee, and place the athlete on crutches.
• If symptoms indicate a tear, refer the athlete to a physician immediately.

Meniscus (Cartilage) Tear

Description

The knee has two cartilages or menisci, the medial (inside) and the lateral (outside). The medial meniscus is more apt to be injured than the lateral and is frequently torn in conjunction with a medial collateral ligament tear. The meniscus tears when the knee twists, usually while the athlete is running or cutting, either with or without a direct collision. The lateral collateral ligament may also be involved in a lateral meniscus tear.

Symptoms

• Immediate and moderately severe pain.
• The athlete is usually unable to fully extend the injured leg and may also complain that the knee "locks" or gets "stuck" during movement.
• Joint line swelling appears within 12 to 24 hours after the injury. Immediate swelling indicates a possible anterior cruciate tear.

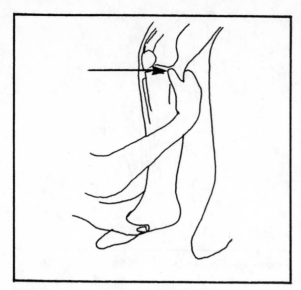

Figure 16-9. Feeling for joint line tenderness

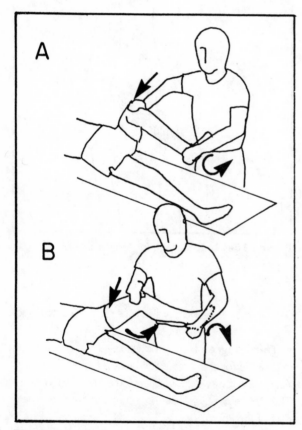

Figure 16-10. Testing for meniscus tears: (A) With leg externally rotated, place valgus stress on knee; (B) Slowly extend leg. If click or pop is felt, torn medial meniscus is suspected.

Exam

- Palpate the joint line for tenderness (Fig. 16-9). This is the most reliable sign of meniscal damage.
- Have the athlete bend his or her knees to about 90 degrees and examine the joint line for swelling.
- Test for meniscal tears in one of the following ways:

  1. The athlete should lie on a table with the injured leg externally rotated. Place valgus stress (pressing inward) on knee (Figure 16-10A).

  2. Place one hand on the injured knee and slowly extend the leg (Figure 16-10B). If you feel a click or a pop, suspect a torn medial meniscus.

Treatment

- Apply ice and a knee wrap and immobilize the knee.
- The athlete should use crutches to avoid putting weight on the injured knee.
- The athlete should see a physician to confirm the diagnosis.

Rehabilitation

- If possible, the athlete should see a physical therapist for a comprehensive program consisting of rehabilitation exercises to strengthen the quadriceps and hamstring muscles and exercises to maintain flexibility of the knee.

Prevention

Athletes should follow preseason and postseason programs for strengthening the hamstring and quadriceps muscles.

Medial and Lateral Collateral Ligament Tears

Description

The collateral ligaments run down either side of the knee, providing stabilization. A direct blow to the lateral (outside) portion of the knee when the foot is planted drives the knee inward, placing stress on the medial collateral ligament. If the blow falls on the medial (inside) portion of the knee, the lateral collateral ligament receives the stress. There are three degrees of ligament tears, progressing from the minor damage of

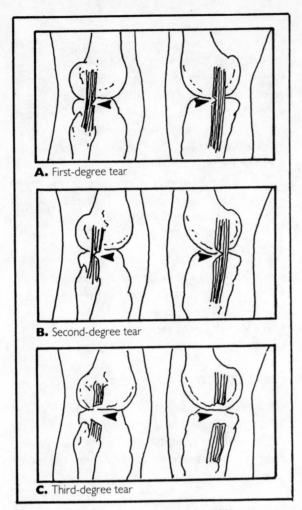

A. First-degree tear

B. Second-degree tear

C. Third-degree tear

Figure 16-11. Medial and lateral collateral ligament tears

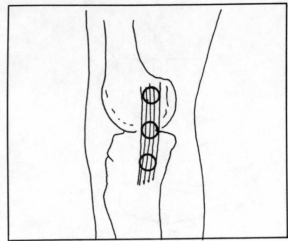

Figure 16-12. Tender sites for torn medial collateral ligament

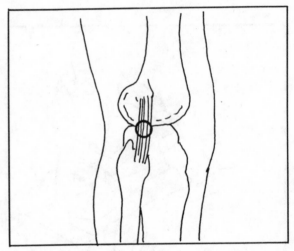

Figure 16-13. Tender site for torn lateral collateral ligament

a first-degree tear to the third-degree tear in which the ligaments are completely torn (Fig. 16-11). The medial collateral ligament has two major components—one superficial and one deep. The superficial component can be torn without damaging the deep component. A deep-component tear is commonly associated with tears of the medial meniscus. Anterior and posterior cruciate ligament tears can also accompany severe medial and lateral collateral ligament tears.

Symptoms

• Pain that accompanies running and cutting characterizes **first-degree** tears. The athlete feels pain but does not feel that the knee is about to give way.
• **Second-degree** tears produce immediate disability. The pain is more intense and the athlete is usually unable to walk without feeling that the knee will give way.

Second-degree tears may also cause some swelling, and it is painful to put weight on the injured leg.
• **Third-degree** tears produce severe pain, making it impossible for the athlete to walk on the injured knee. Any amount of weight will cause the knee to give way. The athlete may feel pain on either the outer or inner part of the knee.

Exam

• Palpate the joint line over the ligament. Figure 16-12 depicts the three sites that may be tender with a torn medial collateral ligament. Keep in mind that tenderness in the joint line can also mean a torn meniscus. Figure

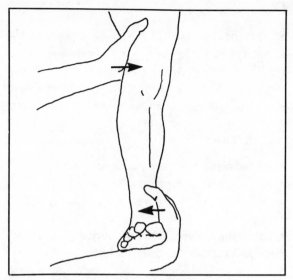

Figure 16-14. Medial collateral ligament stress test

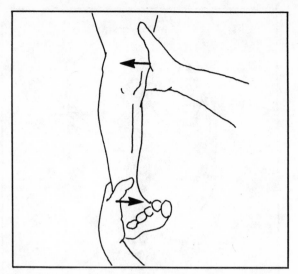

Figure 16-15. Lateral collateral ligament stress test

16-13 shows the area of tenderness for lateral collateral ligament tears.

• Test for stability of the ligaments. To test the medial collateral ligament, place one hand above the ankle joint and the other hand on the outside of the knee pressing inward (valgus stress). Check to see if the knee "opens" medially (Fig. 16-14). If the knee is unstable in full extension, the deep component of the medial collateral ligament is torn. Test the superficial component in the same way, except that the knee should be flexed to 30 degrees.

To test the lateral collateral ligaments, reverse your hand position and press from the inside of the knee to the outside (varus stress). See if the knee "opens" on the outside (Fig. 16-15).

• With **first-degree** tears, stressing the medial collateral ligament causes pain over the ligament, but there is no instability of the joint. **Second-degree** tears produce greater internal pain in reaction to touch and stress. Stressing the knee while it is bent at 30 degrees reveals instability, but the joint regains stability with full extension. **Third-degree** tears have the same characteristics as second-degree tears, except that the knee remains unstable even when fully extended.

NOTE: Always do the same tests on the uninjured knee to compare joint laxity, as some people have normally lax joints.

Treatment

• Apply ice and elevate and immobilize the knee. The athlete should use crutches until he or she can bear weight without pain. First-degree tears usually heal within 7 to 10 days.

• After 24 to 48 hours of P-R-I-C-E and nonsteroidal anti-inflammatories, the athlete can begin putting weight on the injured knee. Sometimes athletes can safely start quadriceps setting exercises less than 48 hours after the injury. When it is no longer painful to put weight on the leg, the athlete should begin exercises to strengthen the quadriceps muscles. He or she can resume full participation once there is no more pain over the ligament and the knee meets all the criteria for returning to activity (see below).

• Second- and third-degree tears require immediate physician evaluation.

Prevention

Rule changes in football have helped prevent many knee injuries. Coaches should enforce blocking and tackling by the rules, and all athletes should follow a preseason and postseason program of strengthening exercises for hamstring and quadriceps muscles.

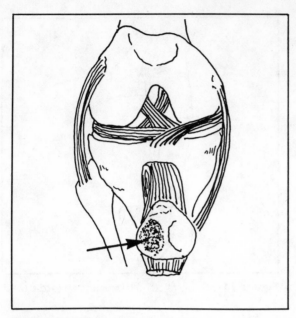

Figure 16-16. Chondromalacia of kneecap

Overuse Injuries

Chondromalacia

(Runner's Knee)

Description

Abnormal movement of the kneecap through the grooves in the lower part of the femur, often the result of a drastic increase in activity, causes pain in the kneecap known as **chondromalacia** (Fig. 16-16). Weakness of the vastus medialis muscle, width of the hips, and flat feet are all factors that contribute to this abnormal tracking, and it is common in sports that involve extensive running.

Symptoms

• Pain in the kneecap, usually described as deep and aching.
• When asked to show the location of the pain, athletes usually point to a spot along the medial (inside) part of the kneecap.
• Walking up and down stairs and sitting with the knee bent for prolonged periods, as in small cars or movie theaters, aggravates the pain.

Exam

• Have the athlete sit with the knee extended and the leg relaxed. Press the kneecap firmly downward against the femoral grooves and ask the athlete to raise the leg (Fig. 16-17). This movement should reproduce the pain.
• Feel for grating or crunching as the kneecap moves.

Treatment

• Ice and nonsteroidal anti-inflammatories.
• A crucial part of the treatment is a program of exercises to strengthen the vastus medialis muscle (see Fig. 16-29).
• Special shoe inserts called **orthotics** can help correct such structural defects as flat feet.
• Rehabilitation exercises should emphasize general quadriceps and vastus medialis strengthening and hamstring stretching.

Prevention

Identify athletes who have a history of knee problems and have them begin knee exercises before an injury occurs.

Jumper's Knee

Description

Jumper's knee is an inflammation of the tendon below the kneecap that results from consistent pounding stress on the knee in such sports as volleyball, basketball, and running.

Symptoms

• Pain below the kneecap, where the patellar tendon attaches to the lower portion of the patella (Fig. 16-18).
• Minimal swelling—a large amount is unusual.
• Pain is intermittent at first but becomes constant and is worse when walking or climbing stairs.
• Jumping, squatting, and cutting also aggravate the pain.

Exam

• Palpate for point tenderness at the site shown in Figure 16-18.

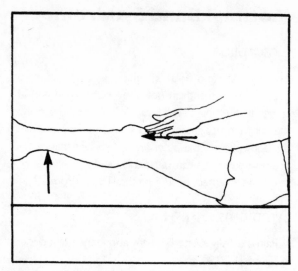

Figure 16-17. Patella compression test

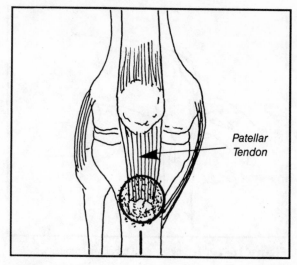

Figure 16-19. Attachment of patellar tendon to tibial tuberosity

Patellar Tendon

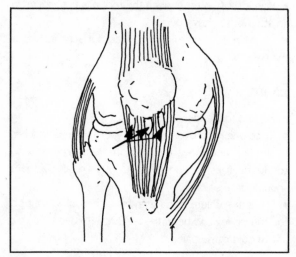

Figure 16-18. Jumper's knee

Treatment

• Ice massage, nonsteroidal anti-inflammatories, and 3 to 4 days of rest.

• A recurring condition may make it necessary to remove an athlete from participation for 2 to 4 weeks before allowing him or her to gradually return to full activity.

Prevention

Avoid heavy weight training with lower extremities. Ease into jumping gradually at the beginning of the season. Encourage athletes to follow an adequate stretching routine before and after activity.

Osgood-Schlatter's Disease

Description

The kneecap (patellar) tendon attaches the kneecap to the lower legbone (tibia) at the tibial tuberosity (Fig. 16-19). This tuberosity is weakened by a child's normal growth spurt between the ages of ten and fifteen, becoming susceptible to small tears produced by the pull of the patellar tendon that occurs with jumping activities, particularly volleyball and basketball.

Symptoms

• Pain and swelling over the tuberosity.

• The pain increases with jumping and running.

Exam

• Palpate for a tender bump (Fig. 16-20).

• Check the quadriceps muscles for weakness. Ask the athlete to extend each leg (as shown in Fig. 16-26) while you resist this extension. Note any difference in strength.

Treatment

• Ice and nonsteroidal anti-inflammatories.

• Exercises to increase flexibility and strength of the quadriceps.

• Severe cases may require the athlete to rest for 1 or 2 weeks before gradually returning to activity.

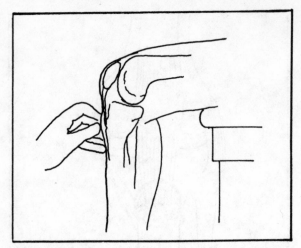

Figure 16-20. Feeling for tibial tuberosity tenderness

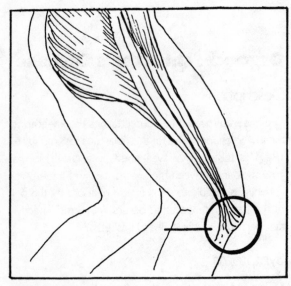

Figure 16-21. Location of iliotibial band

• Refer the athlete to a physician if pain persists longer than 2 weeks.

Prevention

The athlete should wear a knee pad, avoid kneeling, and limit leg extension exercises that use heavy resistance.

Iliotibial Band Syndrome

Description

The iliotibial band (ITB) is a thick band of tissue that extends from the thigh down over the knee and attaches to the tibia (Fig. 16-21). When the knee bends (flexion) and straightens (extension), the ITB slides over the bony parts of the outer knee. Activities that involve prolonged running can cause this band to become irritated and inflamed, producing the ITB syndrome.

Symptoms

• Pain is usually located directly above the point circled in Figure 16-21.
• The athlete may walk with a stiff leg to relieve the pain.
• Pain is most intense when the foot hits the ground in an attempt to slow down.
• Running downhill or on banked surfaces increases the pain.

Exam

• Palpate for tenderness.
• Place one hand over the spot where the ITB attaches to the tibia and move the leg from 90 degrees flexion to 30 degrees flexion (Fig. 16-22). This movement should cause pain.
• Have the athlete stand with his or her full weight on the injured leg and bend the leg 30 to 40 degrees. This also should cause pain.

Treatment

• Ice and nonsteroidal anti-inflammatories
• Decreased activity, particularly in any sports that involve running downhill or on banked surfaces
• Stretching exercises

Prevention

Emphasize proper stretching exercises before and after running. Encourage athletes to return to activity gradually after an injury and to avoid downhill and banked running surfaces.

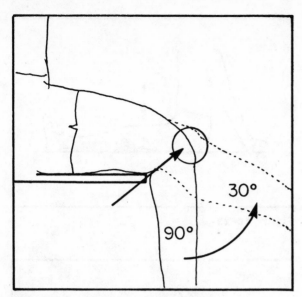

Figure 16-22. Movement of leg produces pain in ITB syndrome

Rehabilitation

Criteria for Returning to Activity

The risk of reinjury greatly increases when an athlete returns to competition too soon. Hurrying through the rehabilitation phase reduces an athlete's overall effectiveness and can lead to permanent damage. The following criteria can be used to determine an athlete's readiness to return to competition following a knee injury:

• The injured knee has regained full range of motion without pain.

• The injured knee has regained normal strength comparable to the uninjured knee.

• The athlete's cardiovascular endurance has returned to normal.

• The injured knee joint has little or no fluid present.

• The athlete is able to pass the following functional tests:

  1. Jog straight ahead without limping

  2. Sprint straight ahead without limping

  3. Do cariocas without "giving in" to the injured knee

  4. Sprint and cut in either direction without favoring the injured knee

  5. Jump on both legs ten times; jump on the injured leg 10 times

Knee Rehabilitation Program

Rehabilitation exercises are vital to the recovery process following an injury and/or surgery to the knee. Muscles lose strength within only a few weeks after an injury, and that strength must be regained before the athlete attempts to return to competition. Though muscles lose strength quickly, the recovery process can take months and can sorely test an athlete's patience. The coach and trainer play an important role in the athlete's rehabilitation, lending guidance (ensuring that the athlete performs the exercises correctly) and moral support (keeping the athlete from becoming discouraged and neglecting or hedging on the prescribed exercises).

An athlete who is facing surgery should strengthen the muscles surrounding the knee prior to the operation. After surgery, the athlete should follow the guidelines established by the physician or physical therapist.

The severity of the knee injury will determine the appropriate exercises for the rehabilitation program. Before initiating any exercise program, consult the athlete's physician or therapist for directions. For the duration of the program, apply moist heat (in the form of either a hot whirlpool or a hydrocollator pack) for 20 minutes before the athlete exercises. Apply ice for 20 minutes following the workout. Any rehabilitation program should be started slowly. If swelling occurs in the knee joint, have the athlete decrease the number of exercises and gradually build up again to the desired amount.

Knee Exercises

Quadriceps Setting

• Sit on the floor and place a couple of rolled-up towels under the affected knee. Slowly push the back of the knee against the towels (Fig. 16-23). You should feel your thigh muscle (quadriceps) tightening and the kneecap moving. Hold the muscle tight for 5 seconds and then relax. Repeat 25 times.

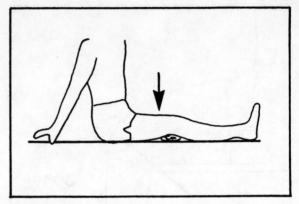

Figure 16-23

Straight Leg Raising

• Lie on your back and, keeping your knee absolutely straight, lift leg to 45 degrees (Fig. 16-24). Lower the leg slowly. Repeat 15 times and then rest. Do 3 sets of 15 repetitions. As your strength increases, drape a gym bag over your ankle to act as a weight.

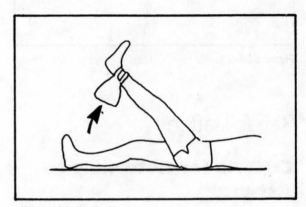

Figure 16-24

Leg Kick

• Stand upright and, keeping the knees absolutely straight, lift the affected leg off the floor (Fig. 16-25). Raise leg up to 45 degrees and slowly lower it. A gym bag can be used for a weight. Repeat 15 times, then rest. Do 3 sets of 15 repetitions.

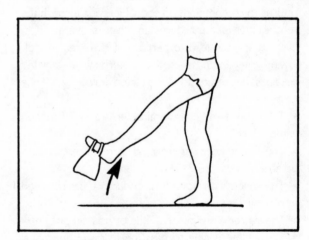

Figure 16-25

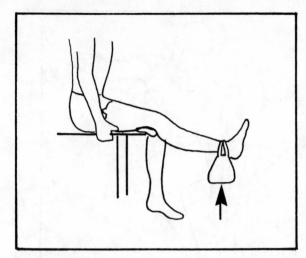

Figure 16-26

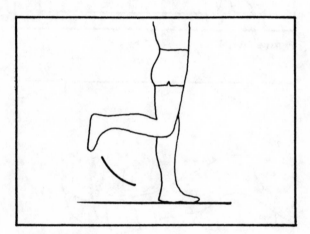

Figure 16-27

Leg Extension

• Sit on a high table with the back of your knee against the edge of the table. A towel can be used for padding. From its bent position, straighten the knee as fully as possible (Fig. 16-26). Hold for 3 seconds. Do 3 sets of 15 repetitions. Add weight, such as a gym bag or purse, as your strength increases. If you notice increased pain or swelling during this exercise, discontinue it and seek advice from your physician.

• A leg extension machine can be used for this exercise. Begin with light weights and progress upward from there. Do one leg at a time. Compare the injured leg to the normal one to determine the maximum weight you can attain. On each repetition, lift the weight slowly until the knee is straight. Hold for 3 seconds and then slowly lower it. Pain and swelling are indications that you are not doing the exercise correctly. Obtain advice from your trainer, doctor, or physical therapist.

Hamstring Curl

• Stand erect and maintain your balance by holding on to a table or another fixed object. Bend the knee by bringing the foot up behind you (Fig. 16-27). A weighted bag can be used to increase resistance. You can also use a weight machine to perform hamstring curls. Use the same precautions given above for leg extensions.

Iliotibial Band Stretch

• This exercise is especially helpful in cases of iliotibial band syndrome. With your injured leg toward the inside, stand sideways to the wall (Fig. 16-28). Place your nearest hand on the wall for support, cross the uninjured leg over the injured one, keeping the foot of the injured leg stable, and lean into the wall. Hold the stretch for 5 seconds and repeat. Do 3 sets of 15 repetitions.

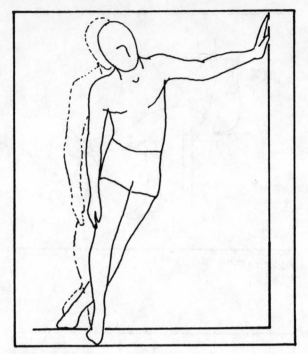

Figure 16-28

Chondromalacia Exercise

• Lie on your back with a rolled-up towel under your knee. Straighten your knee (Fig. 16-29). Move it up and down slowly. A weight can be added. Do 3 sets of 30 repetitions twice daily.

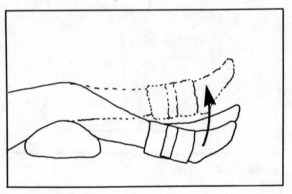

Figure 16-29

Stanley R. Watson

17

Lower Leg
Injuries

This chapter describes injuries to the area below the knee and above the ankle. These injuries include medial tibial stress syndrome (shinsplints and stress fractures), compartment syndromes, and calf muscle tears.

Medial Tibial Stress Syndrome
(Shinsplints)

Description

This injury is usually related to poor training habits, a change in running surface, a new or different style of shoe, or a sudden increase in mileage or in the duration of the workout. It is most commonly seen in poorly conditioned athletes at the beginning of a season, but well-trained athletes who increase their mileage rapidly can also be vulnerable to it.

Shinsplints occur when the muscles and tendons around the shinbone (the tibia) become inflamed and tender. If an athlete continues to exercise, trying to ignore or "run through" the pain, the injury can progress to a more severe form called a **stress fracture**, in which the bone itself is damaged. Both injuries result from small, repetitive stresses that eventually add up to more painful problems. The symptoms, examination, and treatment are identical for both.

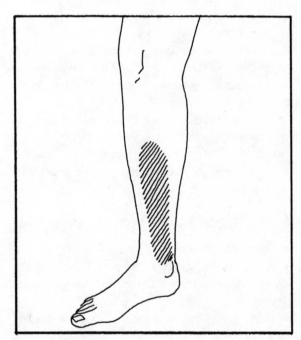

Figure 17-1. Location of pain with shinsplint

Symptoms

• Athlete complains of pain along the lower portion or medial side of the tibia (Fig. 17-1). The pain is often described as deep or throbbing and sometimes as aching.
• Initially the pain occurs at the beginning of the workout and disappears with continued exercise. It then re-

turns 2 to 3 hours after the workout is completed.

• Later the pain may be present before, during, and after exercise. Athletes may alter their gaits, even to the point of limping.

Exam

• Palpate along the lower portion of the shin. Tenderness in response to this pressure is the classic finding in cases of shinsplints. Pain may also be felt in the surrounding tissues, but it is most intense just over the sharp edge of the shin.

• Check for swelling or redness in the same area.

• Test to see if the pain increases when the athlete points the toes downward away from the body or when this motion is resisted (Fig. 17-2).

Treatment

• The best treatment is rest. In addition, complete abstinence from the motions that led to the injury is essential for at least several days.

• If the pain is severe, or if the athlete develops a limp, he or she should use crutches for 2 to 3 days.

• Nonsteroidal agents will reduce both pain and inflammation.

• Well-conditioned athletes, such as long-distance or marathon runners, who develop this syndrome may get good results simply by decreasing their mileage. If the symptoms go away, mileage can be **gradually** increased.

Rehabilitation and Prevention

• Maintain cardiorespiratory fitness.

• When athletes no longer feel tenderness over the lower shin, they are ready to resume running activities. The following routines are recommended:

1. Moist heat applied to the shin for 5 minutes before exercising.

2. Warm-up exercises and calisthenics for 3 to 5 minutes. Then follow with:

3. Heel cord stretch (Fig. 17-3). Keep heels flat on the floor and lean toward a wall. Be far enough away from the wall that you feel the heel cord stretch. Lean toward the wall 5 times with knees straight and 5 times with knees bent. Hold the stretch for 10 to 15 seconds and do not bounce.

4. Gradual progression from walking to jogging to running.

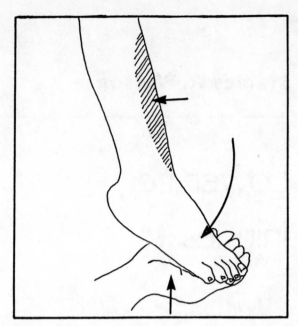

Figure 17-2. Test for shinsplint

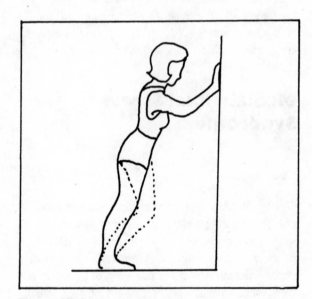

Figure 17-3. Heel cord stretch

5. Ice applied to the affected area for 10 minutes after exercising, **even if there is no pain**.

• Exercise terrain should be changed to a smooth, flat surface and mileage slowly increased over a 2 to 3 week period.

• If the symptoms of this syndrome persist despite an adequate treatment and rehabilitation program, the athlete should be referred to a physician.

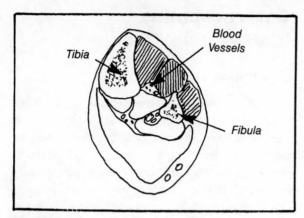

Figure 17-4. Compartment syndromes

Compartment Syndromes

Description

The muscles of the lower leg are enclosed within tight-fitting compartments whose walls are composed of a rigid, inelastic type of tissue. Blood vessels and nerves run through these compartments, and during heavy exercise the muscles expand and put pressure on the nerves and blood vessels. Compartment syndromes occur when muscle pressure cuts off the blood supply to nerves and muscles (Fig. 17-4). This injury is divided into two categories, acute and chronic. The acute injury often afflicts out-of-shape athletes who suddenly begin a heavy program of exercise. A kick in the shin that is followed by swelling can also produce this syndrome. In addition, it can occur in athletes who start training on hilly terrain or in runners whose shoes have an overly flexible sole.

Symptoms

• **Acute**. Athletes complain of severe pain—described as deep, throbbing, crampy, or stabbing—all along lateral side of the lower leg (Fig. 17-5). Immobilization does not lessen the pain. The athlete may complain of abnormal feelings in the foot, such as tingling, numbness, or electricity. Severe cases may result in foot drop, which occurs when swelling is severe enough to cause nerve damage, resulting in the inability to lift the foot off the floor.

• **Chronic**. This form usually involves both legs. During periods of heavy training, athletes may experience pain along the shin or outside of the leg during exercise. The pain is dull and aching but progresses to weakness in the muscles if the athlete continues running.

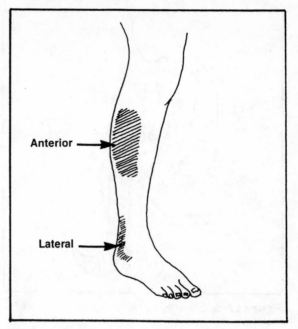

Figure 17-5. Location of pain with compartment syndromes

Exam

• **Acute**. Palpate the leg. The increased pressure may be detectable as increased tension on the surface. The skin may become shiny and warm. Wiggle the athlete's big toe or gently move the foot toward or away from the body (stretch sign) to see if that increases the pain. If the front (anterior) compartment is involved, the athlete may complain of abnormal sensations in the web space between the first two toes. If the outside (lateral) compartment has increased pressure, the top of the foot may be numb or tingly.

• **Chronic**. A chronic condition will usually produce a normal exam result unless the exam is done immediately after a run. Ask the athlete to go out and run to the point of pain and then conduct your exam immediately. This usually reveals pain and swelling over the lateral side of the lower leg. A consulting physician may measure the pressure in these compartments before and after exercise.

Treatment

• If symptoms indicate acute compartment syndrome, the only treatment is rapid referral to a physician. Physicians have a method of measuring pressure in the compartments, and immediate surgery may be required to relieve excessive pressure.

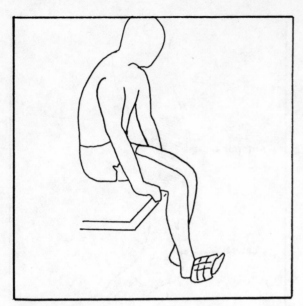

Figure 17-6. Lower leg muscle strengthening

• If symptoms indicate chronic compartment syndrome, a single modification in training technique may relieve the pressure. Athletes should avoid running uphill or running on their toes. Shoes should be checked for excessive flexibility of the sole. Long-distance runners may find that the pain recurs at the same mileage or at the same speed time after time. This can often be avoided by decreasing mileage and/or speed. If symptoms persist despite these measures, referral to a physician is warranted and sometimes surgery is needed.

Rehabilitation

• Stretching and strengthening of the lower leg muscles may relieve or help avoid compartment syndromes (Fig. 17-6).

Prevention

As with other overuse injuries, careful attention to stretching and good training techniques is critical to avoiding injury. It may be helpful to identify athletes who have had previous problems and refer them for possible use of orthotics.

Gastrocnemius (Calf Muscle) Tear

Description

The calf muscle, or **gastrocnemius**, is the large muscle on the back of the lower leg, and it is the one used to raise oneself onto one's toes. A tear may be the result of coming to a quick stop after a hard sprint, running backwards, and sometimes jumping. Usually the athlete is unable to continue to participate. Running, jogging, or even walking can produce severe pain in the calf area. Standing on one's toes is extremely painful with even minor muscle tears. **The pain produced by this injury makes it very frightening for athletes.**

Symptoms

• A tear in the gastrocnemius produces sudden, sharp, burning pain in the calf (Fig. 17-7). Athletes with this injury commonly report feeling as though they have been hit, kicked, or shot in the leg.

Exam

• Gently palpate the muscle to find the most tender area.
• Provide resistance as the athlete pushes the foot down as if pushing on a gas pedal (Fig. 17-8). This reproduces the pain in gastrocnemius tears.

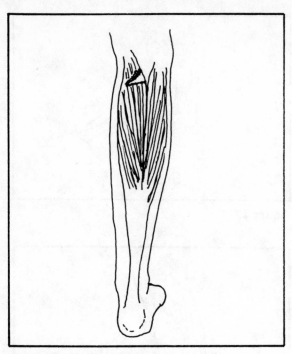

Figure 17-7. Tear in gastrocnemius muscle

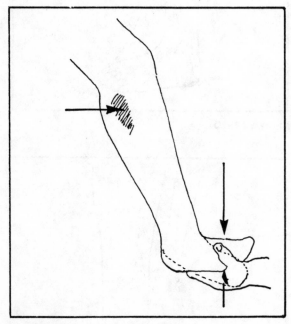

Figure 17-8. Test for gastrocnemius tear

Treatment

• P-R-I-C-E is crucial during the first 48 hours following the injury. The maximum allowable doses of nonsteroidal anti-inflammatory drugs are recommended for the first week.

• Keep injured athletes off their feet, with the lower leg wrapped, iced, and elevated above the level of the heart for the first 48 to 72 hours. This decreases the amount of bleeding into the muscle and speeds recovery.

NOTE: The most important thing to keep in mind about this injury is that early and proper treatment can prevent or lessen the body's inflammatory response.

Rehabilitation

• The duration of an athlete's absence from activity may be greatly reduced by early initiation of therapy and strict adherence to the P-R-I-C-E regimen. Small tears take about 2 weeks to heal. Most athletes can expect to be sidelined for 5 to 6 weeks. Severe tears may require 8 weeks or more to heal.

• The timing of an athlete's return to activity depends on the amount of pain and swelling. Expect the development of bruising down the back of the leg and in the ankle and do not be alarmed by the discoloration. Progression through the following exercises will provide adequate rehabilitation. **Remember: The muscle should be used to the point of discomfort, but not to the point of pain**.

Lower Leg Exercises

Level 1: Gentle Muscle Stretching

• Begin this exercise after 72 hours of P-R-I-C-E therapy. Have the athlete sit in a chair and use a towel to gently pull the foot toward the knee (Fig. 17-9). Gradually apply gentle resistance.

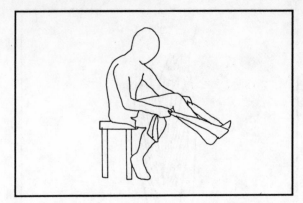

Figure 17-9

Level 2: Two-Legged Toe Raises

• When the towel exercises can be performed repeatedly without pain, the athlete can begin two-legged toe raises (Fig. 17-10). Most of the weight should be borne on the uninjured leg. Begin with repetitions of 10 toe raises and advance slowly from that point.

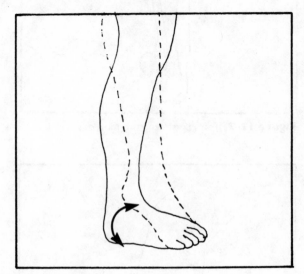

Figure 17-10

• The next step is to increase the stretching effect on the calf muscle by placing a block of wood or a brick under the toes (Fig. 17-11). Always have a handhold nearby for balance.

Level 3: One-Legged Toe Raises

• These can be started once the athlete masters 3 sets of 10 repetitions of the two-legged toe raises. Again, a handhold should be available to provide balance, as the injured muscle will still be very weak. Once the athlete can complete 3 sets of 10 repetitions of one-legged toe raises on each leg with equal smoothness and speed, he or she can begin jogging. After one week of slow jogging, the athlete can gradually move up to running.

NOTE: The athlete should be told that 20 percent of people who incur this injury also tear the same muscle on the opposite leg sometime in the future.

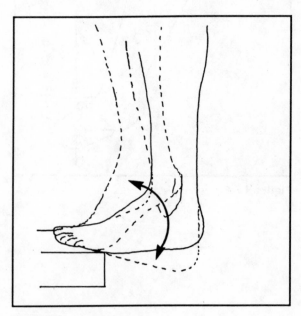

Figure 17-11

Ankle Injuries

Ankle injuries are a major cause of lost playing time in athletics. What athletes commonly call a "twisted" ankle usually consists of damaged ligaments. The most common type of ankle injury results from inverting (turning in) the ankle, which damages one or all of the lateral (outside) ligaments, depending on the severity.

The bones that comprise the ankle (Fig. 18-1) include the **tibia** (shinbone), **fibula** (thin bone next to the shin), **talus**, **navicular**, and **calcaneus** (heel bone). The **deltoid** ligament supports the medial (inside) part of the ankle. The ligaments on the lateral side form a group consisting of the **anterior talofibular, calcanofibular**, and **posterior talofibular** (Fig. 18-2). Their names indicate the two bones to which these ligaments attach (talofibular = talus to fibula).

Bone and Ligament Injuries

Broken Ankle

Description

Depending on how the injury occurs, any bone in the ankle can be broken, but the most commonly broken bone is the fibula. It breaks when the ankle inverts (Fig. 18-3), most often in such sports as volleyball, basketball, and football.

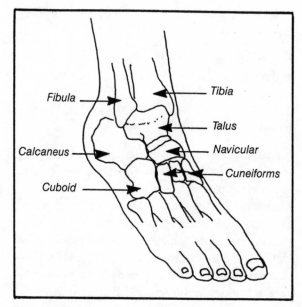

Figure 18-1. Bones of the ankle

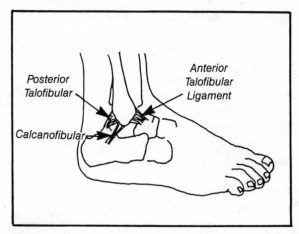

Figure 18-2. Lateral ankle ligaments

119

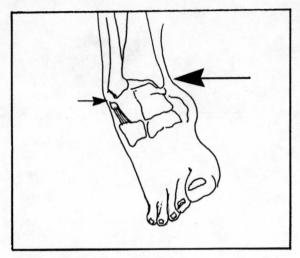

Figure 18-3. Broken ankle bone

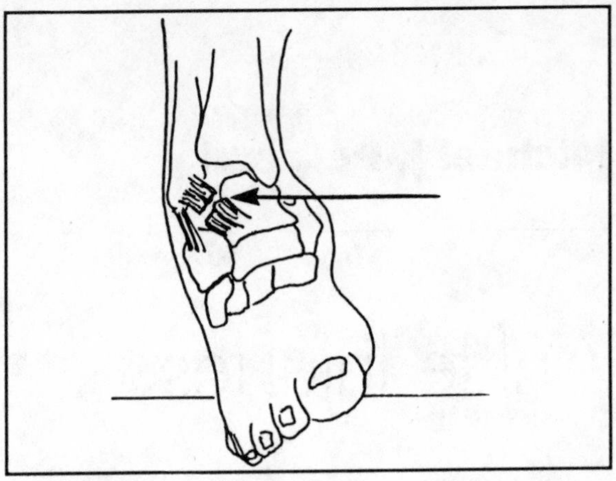

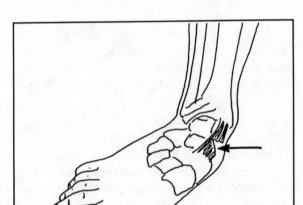

Figure 18-4. Lateral ligament tear

Symptoms

• Pain, particularly when bearing weight.
• Athlete may have heard a "pop" when the ankle turned.

Exam

• Palpate the area, beginning up the leg and working toward the injured area. Examine the whole fibula to rule out multiple breaks.
• Look for swelling and discoloration at the site of injury. Also check below the area of injury.
• Examine the foot. Sometimes a piece is pulled off the foot bone there (see Chapter 19, "Foot Injuries"). **Tenderness directly over any bony area may indicate a broken bone**, although sprains can also produce pinpoint tenderness.
• Check for normal blood flow (skin color) and sensation. This is very important in cases of severe trauma.

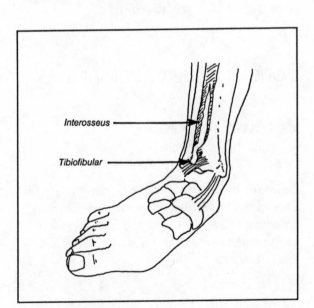

Figure 18-5. Deltoid ligament tear

Treatment

• Immobilize the area with a splint or wrap.
• Elevate the limb and apply ice.
• Refer the athlete to a physician if symptoms indicate a possible broken bone.

Rehabilitation

• The athlete must forcefully rehabilitate the muscles around the ankle before returning to play.

Interosseus

Tibiofibular

Figure 18-6. Other ligament tears

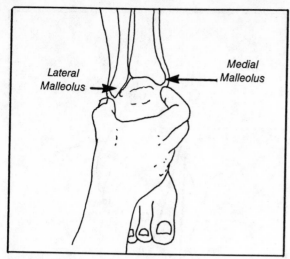

Figure 18-7. Feeling the ankle for tenderness

Prevention

Properly fitting footwear with regulation-length cleats are recommended for field sports. If available, high-top shoes are best for court sports.

Sprained Ankle

Description

Twenty percent of ankle sprains involve the deltoid, interosseous, and tibiofibular ligaments and 80 percent involve the lateral ligaments (anterior talofibular and calcanofibular). A lateral ligament injury is the classic "turned in" ankle, whereas other ligaments are sprained when the ankle is twisted out or in other directions. Lateral ankle injuries are the least serious and have a rapid recovery time. Injuries to the other ligaments are more serious and take longer to heal. Figures 18-4, 18-5, and 18-6 show the locations of these ligamentous tears.

Symptoms

• Knowing what position the foot was in when the injury occurred can help you determine which ligament is torn.
• **Anterior talofibular ligament** sprains occur when the athlete is putting all weight on the toes (plantarflexion).

• **Calcanofibular** sprains occur when the foot is flat but turns inward (inversion) while the athlete is running or walking.
• **Deltoid ligament** sprains can occur when the foot is flat but turned outward and is hit from the lateral side of the leg.
• **Tibiofibular** and **interosseous** sprains occur with twisting movements, such as sliding into base.
• The pain is immediate and may be accompanied by a "pop."
• Swelling begins in 15 to 20 minutes.
• The injured area turns black and blue within a 12-hour period.
• The most severe pain occurs with tibiofibular and interosseous tears.

Exam

• Palpate (touch) over the ankle to ascertain tender ligaments, including the medial and lateral malleolus (Fig. 18-7).
• Evaluate dorsiflexion (Fig. 18-8) and plantarflexion (Fig. 18-9). Limitation of these motions indicates a more severe sprain. Test these motions with and without resistance.
• Do the foot adduction test (Fig. 18-10) with and without resistance. Pain and weakness indicate lateral ligament strains.
• Do the foot abduction test (Fig. 18-11) with and without resistance. Pain and weakness indicate deltoid ligament sprains.
• Using the anterior drawer test (Fig. 18-12), look for tears of the anterior talofibular ligament. Place foot in plantarflexion (toes down). Place one hand on the lower leg and one on the heel. Pull the heel forward while stabilizing the lower leg. Compare the motion with that of the uninjured foot. The test is positive when the heel seems to move forward. Immediately following the injury, pain and spasm may make it difficult to perform the test.
• Check for gross instability, which results when the anterior talofibular and the calcanofibular ligaments are both torn. Place the heel of the foot in the palm of your hand and pull the heel toward you (Fig. 18-13). If the heel is loose, it means that the ligaments are torn.

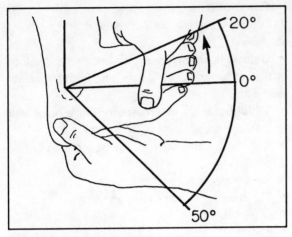

Figure 18-8. Range of ankle dorsiflexion

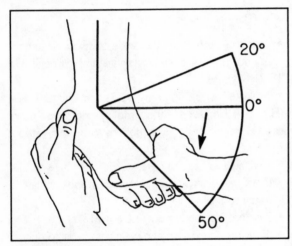

Figure 18-9. Range of ankle plantarflexion

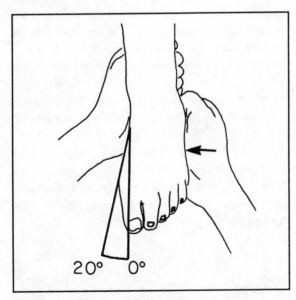

Figure 18-10. Foot adduction test

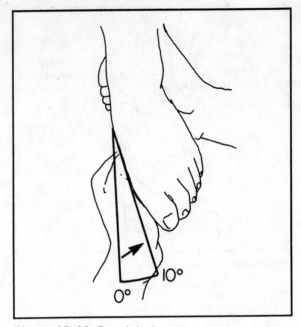

Figure 18-11. Foot abduction test

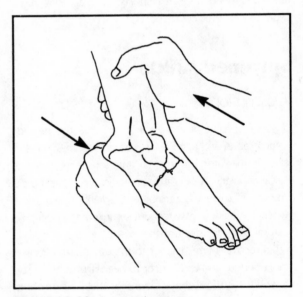

Figure 18-12. Anterior drawer test

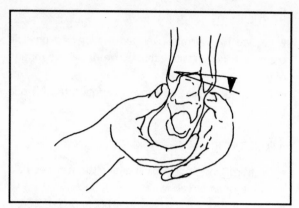
Figure 18-13. Ankle stability test

Ankle sprains are graded 1, 2, or 3, depending on the characteristics revealed by the exam:

Grade 1. Mild pain and swelling, stable joint, normal range of motion, pain-free weight bearing.

Grade 2. Moderate pain and swelling, stable joint, decreased range of motion, and painful weight bearing.

Grade 3. Severe pain and swelling, unstable joint, positive anterior drawer test, painful and limited range of motion, inability to bear weight.

Treatment

• Ice, elevation, and compression.
• Give nonsteroidal anti-inflammatories for both pain and inflammation.
• Have the athlete use crutches and avoid putting weight on the ankle until it is no longer painful.
• Start ankle movement as soon as possible to prevent stiffness. If the athlete can move the foot without pain, begin rehabilitation steps immediately.
• Grade 3 and severe Grade 2 sprains should be evaluated by a physician.

Rehabilitation

• Nonweightbearing movement should begin immediately. Have the athlete lie down with the foot elevated and write the alphabet with the foot 2 to 3 times a day. The ankle should also be dorsiflexed (toes pointing toward the sky) and plantarflexed (toes toward floor) several times a day.
• When the athlete can put weight on the ankle without pain, he or she should begin walking and performing the exercises listed at the end of this chapter. The exercises should be followed with 5 to 10 minutes of ice to decrease swelling.

Prevention

The ankle can be protected by using properly fitting footwear, regulation-length cleats, and high-top shoes if available.

NOTE: Chronic problems can develop from ankle injuries that have received improper or inadequate care. An athlete with a significant sprain (unable to bear weight or "cut" without pain) should never reenter a game. The public has come to expect athletes, particularly professionals, to "play hurt," but this is inappropriate, especially for junior or senior high school athletes. All athletes must be able to run, cut, and land on the ankle without pain. Both ankles should be nearly equal in strength.

Tendon Injuries

Spasm/Dislocation of Peroneal Tendons

Description

The peroneal tendons cross the ankles around the lateral prominence (lateral malleolus) of the ankle. Sometimes, when an athlete inverts (turns in) an ankle, these tendons go into spasm. If the trauma is more severe, the tendons can become dislocated from their attachments. This injury is common in such sports as volleyball, basketball, and football.

Symptoms

• **Spasm**: Pain behind the malleolus, making walking difficult
• **Dislocation**: Severe pain, swelling

Exam

• Check to see if the athlete has difficulty everting (turning out) the ankle, which may indicate a dislocation.
• Palpate for pain over the peroneal tendons (Fig. 18-14).

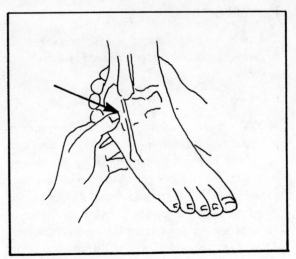

Figure 18-14. Feeling for pain over the peroneal tendons

Treatment

• Spasms subside quickly after application of ice, and there is no subsequent pain. After the spasm resolves, the athlete can return to activity.
• A dislocation requires physician referral. Surgery may be needed.

Peroneal Tendinitis

Description

Peroneal tendons are also subject to overuse, particularly in running sports, gymnastics, and dancing.

Symptoms

• Pain behind the lateral malleolus that develops over time.

Exam

• Palpate for warmth over the tendon and possible crepitus (grinding) with either active or passive motion of the ankle.
• Check for decreased range of motion (ROM) due to pain.

Treatment

• Rest, ice, and nonsteroidal anti-inflammatories help reduce pain and swelling.
• The athlete's training program should be reduced, if not completely stopped, for 3 to 5 days.

Rehabilitation

• Have the athlete perform strengthening exercises as soon as the pain is gone (see below).
• After the pain and swelling subside, the athlete can begin a gradual return to activity.

Prevention

As with most overuse injuries, training errors are the leading cause of peroneal tendinitis. These errors include a sudden increase in running distance or speed or sharp increases in the amount of time spent working out in gymnastics or dancing. Muscle imbalance or overworn shoes can also contribute to this type of injury.

Ankle Exercises

Heel Raises

• Stand with feet flat on floor and then slowly raise yourself up on your toes. Do this with feet in three positions: toes pointed straight ahead, toes pointed in, and toes pointed out (Fig. 18-15). Repeat 30 times each, 3 times a day.

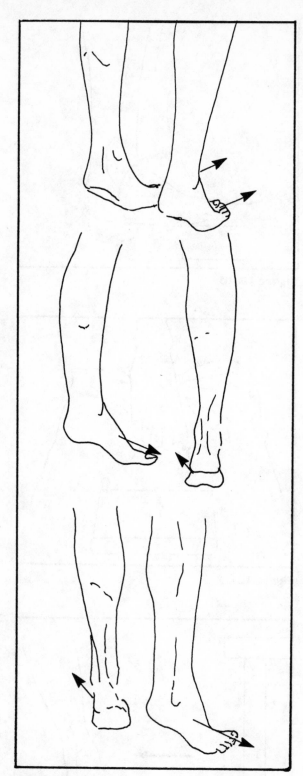

Figure 18-15

Toe Raises

• Stand on a step with heels extending over the edge, drop heels below step, then raise up on toes (Fig. 18-16). Repeat 30 times, 3 times a day.

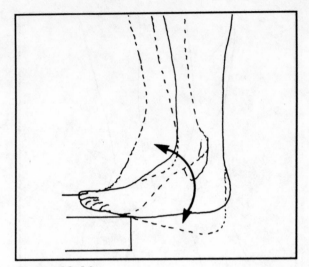

Figure 18-16

Towel Pull

• Sit in a chair and place a towel on the floor in front of you. Use the toes of the injured foot to pull the towel toward you, keeping the heel on the floor. Straighten out the towel and repeat 10 to 15 times twice a day. Also pull towel to right and left. For resistance place a large book on the towel (Fig. 18-17).

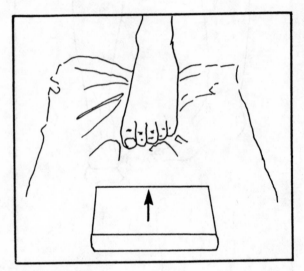

Figure 18-17

Resistance Exercises with Tubing

• Sit and attach one end of some rubber tubing to a heavy object such as a chair or table. Loop the other end around the injured foot. Pull with your foot against the resistance of the tubing through a full range of motion—up, down, in, and out. Do 20 times, 3 times a day (Fig. 18-18).

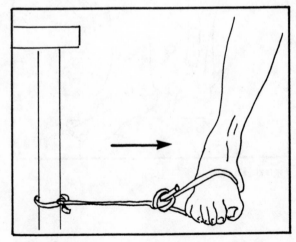

Figure 18-18

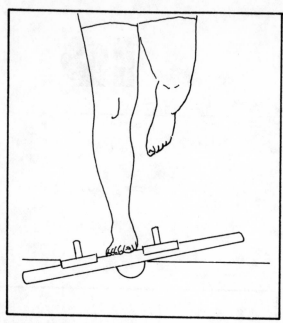

Figure 18-19

NOTE: If an athlete begins limping, all running should be curtailed.

Proprioception

• It is important for the ankle to regain the sense of position (**proprioception**) it loses after injury. Proprioception boards (Fig. 18-19) can be purchased or made. To use the board, the athlete stands on one foot on it and goes through range of motion exercises. This exercise can be repeated 10 times twice a day.

Hopping Exercise

• Hop as high as possible, first on the good leg and then on the injured leg. Hop 10 to 15 times on each leg.

• When athletes can perform the hopping exercise equally well and without pain on both legs, they should begin the exercises in the following section.

Returning to Competition

• Active jogging and walking with ankle taped. Use the following schedule:

   1. Alternately walk 25 yards and jog 25 yards for one mile.

   2. Alternately walk 25 yards and jog 50 yards for one mile.

   3. Alternately walk 25 yards and jog 75 yards for one mile.

   4. Alternately walk 25 yards and jog 100 yards for one mile.

   5. Jog one mile, then increase by a quarter-mile daily to a total distance of three miles.

   6. Repeat steps 1 through 5 at half speed. Do not cut or go in circles; run straight ahead.

   7. Repeat steps 1 through 5 at three-quarters speed, straight ahead.

   8. Repeat steps 1 through 5 at full speed, straight ahead.

• When athletes can sprint at full speed and without a limp, then have them run in circles, both clockwise and counterclockwise. Start with large circles and work down in size.

• When athletes can run the circles at full speed without a limp or pain, have them run figure eights.

• When athletes can run figure eights at full speed without a limp or pain, have them run a zig-zag course the length of a football field.

• Finally, test athletes on right-angle quick-cuts to the right and left. When they can do this, they are ready to return to practice and competition. Make sure they have not lost cardiovascular conditioning.

Michael J. Petrizzi

19

Foot Injuries

The foot is an amazing combination of bones (7 tarsals, 15 metatarsals, 14 phalanges, and 2 sesamoids), ligaments, muscles, and tendons (Fig. 19-1). It must be strong enough to support body weight and absorb the impact of landing after a jump, yet flexible enough to propel the body forward. Injuries to the foot can be traumatic (fractures) or chronic (overuse injuries). Although some foot injuries may not appear disabling, it is very difficult for athletes to compete at their best when it hurts just to walk.

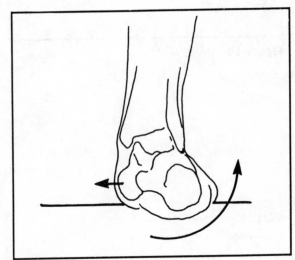

Figure 19-2. Pronation

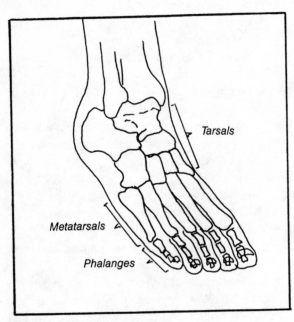

Figure 19-1. Bones of the foot

Many chronic foot injuries are associated with excessive degrees of a foot's normal motions, **pronation** and **supination**. In pronation, the foot "flattens out" and the bones become "looser" in order to adapt to the ground surface or to other stresses. In supination, the foot becomes more rigid, enabling it to act as a lever for "pushing off." However, the foot can often be excessively pronated (too flattened out) while weight bearing (Fig. 19-2). It is therefore important to examine the foot while the athlete is standing. Also look at shoewear patterns (Fig. 19-3). If an athlete hyperpronates, injuries may be helped (or prevented) by shoes designed to resist pronation. Orthotics (arch supports) can also help hyperpronation.

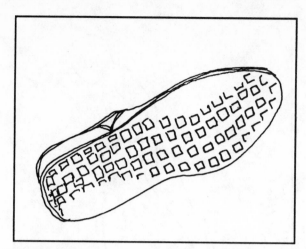

Figure 19-3. Hyperpronation shoewear pattern

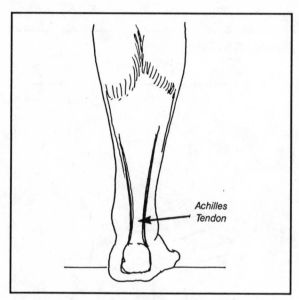

Figure 19-4. Location of Achilles tendon

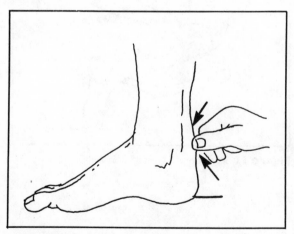

Figure 19-5. Pain over Achilles tendon

Heel Injuries

Achilles Tendinitis

(Heel Pain)

Description

The Achilles tendon connects the calf muscles to the heel (Fig. 19-4). Tight calf muscles can lead to tendon inflammation, as can sudden increases in mileage or speedwork. High-arched feet, shoes with inadequate heel support, and hyperpronation also increase the risk of tendinitis.

Symptoms

• Pain at the top of the heel in back of the foot.
• Pain is aggravated by activity, being worse at the beginning of activity and improving with warm-up.

Exam

• Determine if the athlete is experiencing pain over the Achilles tendon (Fig. 19-5).
• Feel for thickening or a nodule in the tendon.
• Check for decreased ability to raise the foot upward (dorsiflexion), compared with the other foot.

Treatment

• Apply ice to decrease inflammation and pain. Give nonsteroidal anti-inflammatories at maximum dosage for 7 to 10 days.
• The athlete should curtail or discontinue activity until he or she feels no more pain either walking or at rest.
• Elevate the heel by placing heel cups, pads, and wedges in shoes.
• Emphasize adequate stretching of calf muscles before and after workouts. A good calf muscle stretching exercise is shown in Figure 19-6. Stand upright with one foot in front of the other. Keeping the heel of the rear foot on the floor, lean forward and hold the stretch to a count of 10.

Ruptured Achilles Tendon

(Torn Heel Cord)

Description

The Achilles tendon ruptures near the site of its insertion into the calcaneus. Such an injury occurs when the tendon is stretched. Fortunately, this injury is rare in younger athletes, but many physicians caution that an athlete with chronic Achilles tendinitis is at higher risk for a ruptured tendon.

Symptoms

• Same symptoms as those listed above for Achilles tendinitis.
• Sudden, extreme pain in the back of the leg, accompanied by swelling.
• The athlete may claim to have heard a popping or cracking noise at the moment of injury.
• Athlete has difficulty walking and pushing down with the foot.

Exam

• **Thompson test**. With the injured leg placed as shown in Figure 19-7, squeeze the calf muscle. Compare the movement of one leg to the other. If the tendon is ruptured, there will be little or no movement of the foot.
• Also feel over the tendon for a tender area with a palpable gap.

Treatment

• Apply ice to reduce swelling and refer the athlete to a physician.

Prevention

Avoid activity during cases of Achilles tendinitis. Emphasize adequate calf-stretching exercises.

Sever's Disease

(Heel Pain in Children)

Description

This condition occurs in physically active children between the ages of eight and thirteen. It is an inflamma-

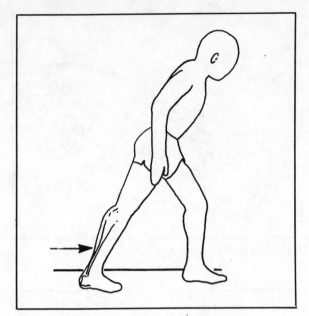

Figure 19-6. Calf muscle stretch

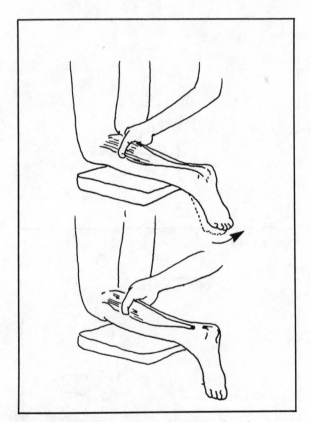

Figure 19-7. Thompson test for torn heel cord

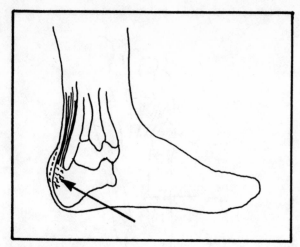

Figure 19-8. Location of Sever's disease

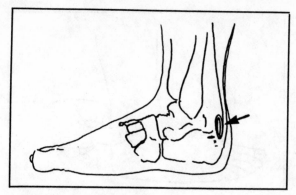

Figure 19-9. Retrocalcaneal bursa

tion of the bone at the point where the heel cord attaches to the calcaneus (Fig. 19-8) and is caused by tension on the heel cord created by tight calf muscles. As children grow older, their bones harden and this condition subsides.

Symptoms

• Athlete feels pain in the back of the heel while running and exercising.
• Wearing shoes may be painful.

Exam

• Look for swelling and tenderness at the site of Achilles tendon insertion.
• Check for decreased dorsiflexion (upward movement) of the injured foot compared to the other foot.

Treatment

• Decrease activity and apply ice.
• Give nonsteroidal anti-inflammatories.
• Use heel lifts and heel pads.
• **Do not do exercises for stretching the heel cord, as these will worsen the condition.**

Retrocalcaneal Bursitis

(Pain behind the Heel Bone)

Description

The retrocalcaneal bursa is a fluid-filled sac lying between the tendon and the heel that helps tendons move over bony areas more efficiently (Fig. 19-9). Chronic irritation of this bursa can lead to swelling and pain.

Symptoms

• Pain at back of heel.
• Other symptoms resemble those of Achilles tendinitis.

Exam

• Feel for tenderness, swelling, and fullness in the area directly in front of the Achilles tendon. Apply pressure in front of the tendon above the point of its insertion into the calcaneus (Fig. 19-10).

NOTE: It is important to distinguish bursitis from Achilles tendinitis.

Treatment

• Same as for Achilles tendinitis.

Prevention

Have the athlete wear adequately padded heel contours in shoes.

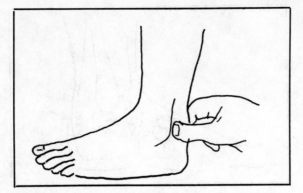

Figure 19-10. Pain area for retrocalcaneal bursitis

Plantar Fasciitis

("Heel Spur" Syndrome)

Description

The plantar fascia is a collection of connective tissue originating at the bottom of the heel and progressing forward toward the ball of the foot (Fig. 19-11). It helps maintain the arch. Plantar fasciitis is painful swelling of this connective tissue. Feet that pronate (flatten out) excessively are most commonly afflicted with this ailment.

Symptoms

• Pain, often disabling, at the base (bottom) of the heel. The pain is usually worse right after taking the first steps in the morning or after sitting and at the beginning of a run. It feels like electricity going through the bottom of the foot.

Exam

• Feel for tenderness over the arch and bottom of the heel (Fig. 19-12).
• Try passive stretching of the fascia by dorsiflexing (raising up) the toes while keeping the heel fixed to see if this worsens the pain.

Treatment

• Athlete should observe a significant decrease in activity or total rest.
• Apply ice and give nonsteroidal anti-inflammatories at maximum dosage.
• A running shoe with excellent heel support may help alleviate the pain.

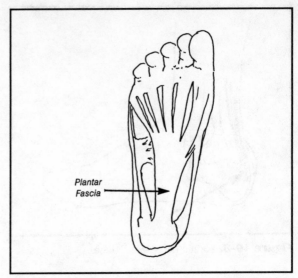

Figure 19-11. Location of the plantar fascia

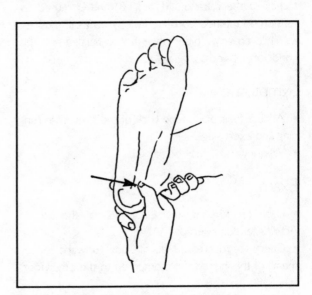

Figure 19-12. Tenderness at bottom of heel

• Plastic heel cups and arch supports may help hyperpronators.
• Running shoes must be worn for every step, including trips to the bathroom in the middle of the night. This injury often takes weeks (and sometimes months) to improve.
• Perform the exercise shown in Figure 19-13. Stand with one foot in front of the other. Keep the rear foot flat and bend the front knee forward. Hold for 5 seconds and repeat 10 times.
• The fascia can also be stretched by rolling the foot on top of a rolling pin.

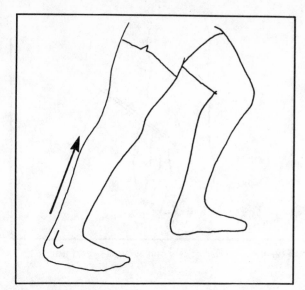

Figure 19-13. Plantar fascia stretch

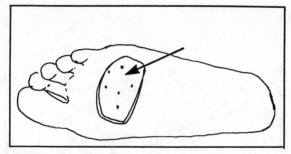

Figure 19-14. Metatarsal pad

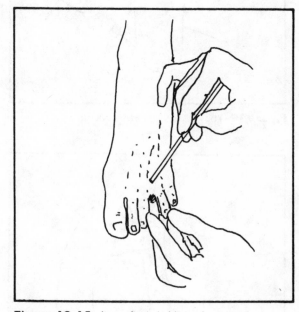

Figure 19-15. Area of pain in Morton's neuroma

Forefoot Injuries

Metatarsalgia

Pain in the ball of the foot is called metatarsalgia. It is often caused by a change in activity, running surface, or shoes. A metatarsal pad (Fig. 19-14) placed behind the painful area is usually all that is needed to relieve the symptoms. Orthotics or special shoes to prevent hyperpronation also help. If there is no improvement after these measures, then consider other causes such as stress fractures and neuromas (described below).

Morton's Neuroma

Description

A neuroma is swelling in a portion of a nerve. It usually affects the nerves between the third and fourth toes or the second and third toes (Fig. 19-15). The nerve irritation results from pressure caused by bones being pushed together. Tight shoes are one possible cause.

Symptoms

• Pain between the second and third toes.
• A tingling, burning feeling extends out to the involved toes.
• Pain increases with walking and weight bearing.

Exam

• Compress foot by applying pressure from both sides—this should reproduce the pain.
• Palpate for pain between the metatarsal bones (Fig. 19-16).

Treatment

• Switch to wider, softer shoes.
• Use a metatarsal pad and avoid jumping on the ball of the foot or on hard surfaces.
• Neuromas may sometimes require surgery. An athlete whose condition does not improve should be referred to a physician.

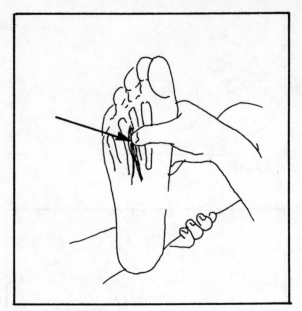

Figure 19-16. Feeling for Morton's neuroma

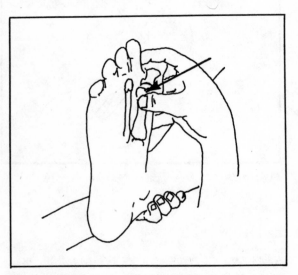

Figure 19-17. Feeling for sesamoid fractures

Sesamoiditis and Sesamoid Stress Fracture

Description

The sesamoid bones are two pea-sized bones located in the tendon that flexes the big toe. They are located on the ball of the foot at the big toe. Repetitive stress can cause them to become inflamed, particularly in such sports as gymnastics, tennis, volleyball, and basketball.

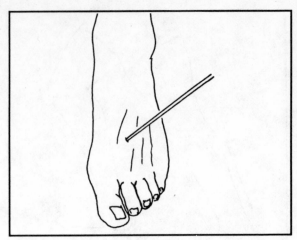

Figure 19-18. Location of metatarsal stress fracture

Symptoms

• Pain under ball of foot at the big toe.

Exam

• Palpate the involved sesamoid under the head of the first metatarsal (Fig. 19-17) to see if this causes pain.
• Check also to see if dorsal (top) and plantar (under-surface) flexion of the great toe while palpating the bone causes pain.

Treatment

• Rest and nonsteroidal anti-inflammatories.
• Padding must be placed behind head of first metatarsal to reduce stress on the sesamoids. Keeping the great toe plantarflexed with tape can also be helpful.

Prevention

Make sure there is adequate padding in shoe.

Metatarsal Stress Fracture

Description

Stress fractures can be caused by a sudden increase in training or a structural defect such as excessive pronation. Athletes participating in running sports, volleyball, or basketball are particularly susceptible.

Symptoms

• Pain in metatarsal, possibly with swelling.

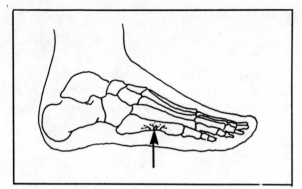

Figure 19-19. Jones fracture

Exam

• Palpate for point tenderness over involved area of metatarsal (Fig. 19-18).
• Examine for small amounts of swelling, usually in the shaft or long part of the bone.

Treatment

• Refer athlete to a physician for evaluation.

Jones Fracture

Description

Often mistakenly used to describe an avulsion fracture (pulled-off piece) of the fifth metatarsal, this term actually means a stress fracture of the middle part of the fifth metatarsal (Fig. 19-19). Symptoms may appear only after an inversion injury (twisting of the ankle).

Symptoms

• Pain in fifth metatarsal, possibly with swelling.

Exam

• Palpate for point tenderness in the fifth metatarsal, **in the proximal third of the bone but not at the base**. Tenderness over the bone in the shaft of a metatarsal is likely to indicate a fracture (Fig. 19-20).

Treatment

• If symptoms indicate a possible fracture, refer the athlete to a physician. Failure of the bone to heal properly can lead to **permanent disability**.

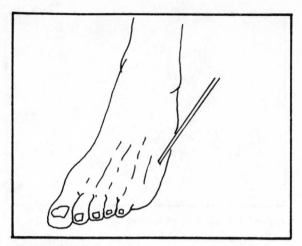

Figure 19-20. Area of pain in Jones fracture

Prevention

Follow a thoughtful training routine. Orthotics can correct certain structural defects in the foot.

Avulsion Fracture of the Fifth Metatarsal

Description

The same conditions that cause a lateral (outside) sprain can lead to an avulsion fracture of the fifth metatarsal. The muscle called the **peroneus brevis** is attached to the base of that bone and, if it is stretched hard enough, may avulse the bone.

Symptoms

• Pain and swelling at the base of the fifth metatarsal.

Exam

• Palpate for point tenderness at base, or **styloid process**, of fifth metatarsal (Fig. 19-21).

Treatment

• If symptoms indicate a fracture, refer the athlete to a physician. The physician may recommend simple strapping and perhaps a splint to limit inversion. These fractures tend to heal well.

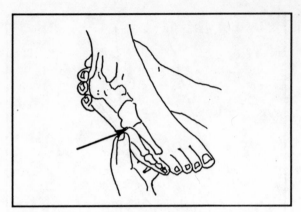

Figure 19-21. Base of fifth metatarsal

Phalanges (Toe) Injuries

Fractured Phalanx

(Broken Toe)

Description

Toes can be broken when they are stepped on or when a heavy object falls on them, or when they are forced backward by direct trauma. As with broken fingers, broken toes can be moved.

Symptoms

• Immediate pain and swelling, discoloration, and possible deformity.

Exam

• Palpate above and below area of tenderness. If the area of maximal tenderness is well localized, this usually indicates a fracture.
• Look for any deformities, particularly while athlete wiggles his or her toes.

Treatment

• If no deformity is evident, all the joints move freely, and only the distal phalanx (tip of the toe) is tender, buddy taping the injured toe to its neighbor may suffice. Be sure to place a small piece of foam between the toes before taping to reduce the chance of skin breakdown.
• It may be necessary to refer the athlete to a physician to see if the bone is broken.

Turf Toe

Description

Turf toe is caused by a hyperextension or dorsiflexion (bending upwards) of the toe(s), which results in strained ligaments. This injury may occur more often these days because of the extreme flexibility of the newer athletic shoes.

Symptoms

• Pain when toeing off (stepping forward) or landing on toes.

Exam

• Palpate for tenderness along plantar (undersurface) ligaments.
• See if the pain is made worse by passively dorsiflexing (bending up) the involved toe(s).

Treatment

• Ice and nonsteroidal anti-inflammatories at maximum dose; buddy taping of toes.
• Place a stiff (possibly metal) insert under the toes and extending all the way to the balls of the feet to decrease the likelihood of aggravating the injury. This injury can take many weeks to heal completely.

Prevention

Consider wearing stiffer, more supportive shoes.

Ingrown Toenails

The big toe can become red and tender along the line of the nail and the skin. This can be a very painful and disabling condition, but it can be prevented by wearing shoes that are not too tight at the tips. Treatment consists of warm soaks, loose shoes, and time. If these simple measures do not help, then physician referral is indicated.

Section 3

Related
Health
Issues

Edward J. Shahady

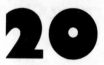

Cheerleaders as Athletes

Because it did not originate as an athletic event, cheerleading has yet to be accepted as an organized sport with its participants treated as athletes. **But cheerleading has become much more than a matter of leading cheers and whipping up enthusiasm for the school team. It has developed into a sophisticated cross between gymnastics and dancing that requires strength and endurance**. Backflips, human pyramids, tumbling routines, and choreographed dancing, taught and supported by summer camps, competitions, and four national organizations—this is cheerleading in the late twentieth century. We would never think of having dancers or gymnasts perform maneuvers similar to those done by cheerleaders without benefit of coaches, trainers, mats, safety equipment, and rules.

The number of injuries to cheerleaders increases yearly. There are an estimated 600,000 cheerleaders in the United States, and each year they sustain over 7,000 injuries that require treatment in emergency rooms. Strains, sprains, and fractures involving ankles, knees, and wrists are the most common injuries, an injury profile similar to that of gymnasts. Serious injuries have become more commonplace. In 1986 a cheerleader died of a head injury after falling from a three-person pyramid; two more were paralyzed, one from a backflip off a minitrampoline and the other from a fall off a pyramid. All three accidents involved college cheerleaders, which is significant because high school athletes emulate college athletes.

The consequence of these serious incidents should not be the imposition of a ban on pyramids and minitrampolines, but rather an increased awareness of the need to make proper conditioning and training, along with safe equipment and rules, an integral part of cheerleading. The selection of a cheerleader can no longer be based on popularity contests or the physical attractiveness of the candidate. Although these may be important attributes, they must be counted as secondary to athletic ability.

Cheerleading practices need to include weight training, flexibility exercises, and warm-up and cool-down routines just like other team practices. Preparticipation evaluation of cheerleaders should be identical to other athletic exams. As outlined in Chapter 30, "Preparticipation Evaluations," the orthopedic evaluation is the most important. The 12-minute run can also be a good way to discover who is in condition and who is not.

Because cheerleading is a sport that requires power and flexibility, training should stress strengthening exercises for quadriceps, hamstrings, biceps, wrists, and adductor muscles as well as maximum flexibility in these muscle groups. Chapters 13, 15, and 16 include exercises for strengthening these muscles.

The North Carolina High School Athletic Association has published the following suggested guidelines for cheerleading:

Recommended Guidelines Governing Cheerleading Safety

1. A comprehensive conditioning program shall be adopted by all cheerleading squads. Emphasis must be placed on problem areas (i.e., leg flexibility, upper arm strength, ankle and wrist strength, etc.).

2. Preceding all practice sessions and performance there shall be structured stretching exercises and a basic warm-up of cheerleading gymnastics (jumps, partner stunts, pyramids, tumbling, etc.).

3. All cheers, chants, dances, or spirit-raising activities shall be **well planned, practiced, and organized to promote the safety of students participating in cheerleading activities**.

4. All squads shall be supervised by a cheerleading coach, sponsor, or other responsible adult during all warm-ups, practices, and performances.

   a. Locations of practices should be suitable for the activities of cheerleaders (i.e., tumbling mats, distance from excessive noise and distractions, etc.).

   b. Practices should also be conducted in an atmosphere conducive to maximum concentration and with minimal talking.

5. **Cheerleading coaches/sponsors should have a background in cheerleading, dance choreography, and/or gymnastics**, and must be knowledgeable in proper cheerleading techniques and safety procedures. Coaches must coach only within their level of expertise and the abilities of their squads. It is recommended that cheerleading coaches/sponsors should regularly attend cheerleading camps and state and local cheerleading clinics to be more knowledgeable in current cheerleading techniques and safety procedures.

6. Sponsors/coaches must know their squad's ability level and must limit the squad's activities accordingly. As quoted from Universal Sports Camp, Inc., "Ability level refers to the squad's talents as a whole, and individuals **should not** be pressed to perform activities until safely perfected." (All routines, pyramids, stunts, and gymnastics shall be practiced to perfection prior to actual performance.)

7. Cheerleaders shall adapt their routines to the environmental conditions and playing surfaces for which stunts, pyramids, and routines are used (i.e., no mount or gymnastics should be done during rain or on slippery surfaces; hot and humid weather may also present problems).

8. Pyramids and partner stunts may be part of the squad's routine, provided the following safety precautions are taken:

   a. No pyramid or stunt formation is to be higher than two levels (see "Mounting Height Defined" below).

   b. No base should support more than 1½ people.

   c. No free roll-offs or free flips off pyramids or stunts.

   d. No knee drops.

   e. No collapsing pyramids or stunts (does not mean cradling).

   f. No toe pitches.

   g. No single support split catch.

   h. Spotters should be present throughout the mounting, result, and dismounting stages of pyramids. (Spotters should always be in position throughout with hands up and eyes on the top mount.)

   i. Back dismounts into a cradle must be received by at least two people (e.g., fireman's catch).

   j. A basket toss is allowed if there is one spotter in back to spot the head along with the two bases.

9. Gymnastic maneuvers where competency has been mastered are permitted. (Coaches/sponsors not knowledgeable in gymnastics should consult someone with expertise in this area to advise them of the ability level of their squad members.)

10. Minitramps, springboards, and similar equipment are prohibited.

11. No jewelry should be worn during practices or performances.

12. Aerobic-type shoes shall be worn.

13. Cheerleaders shall have access to the school athletic trainer and team physician.

14. Cheerleaders shall have a medical examination prior to tryouts, practice, or participation on a squad. Any known medical condition which might interfere with active participation (i.e., asthma, heart condition, epilepsy, diabetes, etc.) should be recorded (see NCHSAA Handbook).

15. A cheerleader who misses practice at which the squad masters a pyramid, stunt, or gymnastics maneu-

ver shall not perform any of those maneuvers at the next performance.

16. Cheerleaders shall travel together and use transportation which has been approved by the school administration.

17. These safety guidelines also apply to practice, game situations, and outside competitions.

18. We recommend that the cheerleading squad be chosen by someone knowledgeable of the skills required.

Rules for Cheerleading Safety: Definition of Terms

Base. The ground level or bottom person of a partner stunt. This person supports the full or partial weight of another person.

Basket Toss. A cheerleading stunt consisting of bases, a top mount, and a spotter. The top stands on the interlocked wrists of the bases. In a coordinated count, the bases dip the legs and throw by extending the arms upward. The top mount rides the throw performing a toe touch. The bases catch the top in a cradle while the spotter supports the head.

Cartwheel. A slow, lateral handspring with arms and legs extended.

Chant. Repetitive words or phrases which may be combined with simple motions, clapping, or a similar beat, to generate a unified crowd response during or between play.

Cheer. An organization and coordination of words and motions which is generally performed by a cheerleading team to draw a unified response from a crowd while play has been stopped.

Collapsing Pyramid. A pyramid in which all persons simultaneously fall or drop so that the top people land on the bottom people in a compact, lying position (see definition of a pyramid).

Cradle. The catching of a dismounting individual with both arms equal and slightly bent.

Dance Routine. Rehearsed, choreographed movements done to music.

Fireman's Catch. The same as cradle but involves more than one person and they must be facing each other. The third person must be in a position to support the head and shoulders.

Dive Forward Roll. A forward roll initiated from a running or standing position. The person performing the dive roll punches off by leaping forward, out-

stretches arms, and tucks quickly to perform a forward revolution on the ground.

Flip. A dismount from a pyramid or partner stunt in which the person flipping performs an unassisted backward or forward full rotation to land on the floor or in a cradle.

Front or Back Tuck. The body turns forward or backward in a full circle from a standing position and lands in a standing position. A front or back tuck is a flip performed by an individual on ground level.

Forward Roll or Somersault. A roll initiated from a squatting position on the ground, in which a person turns forward or backward in a complete revolution in a tucked position and finally lands on the feet.

Handspring. A gymnastic maneuver in which the body turns forward or backward in a full circle from a standing position, and lands first on the hands and finally on the feet.

Handstand. The act of supporting the body on the hands with the trunk and legs balanced in the air.

Jump. To spring from the ground by the muscular action of the feet and legs.

Knee Drop. Jumping into a kneeling position on the floor or ground by bending both knees simultaneously and landing on the knees and skin area of the leg. The individual goes directly from a standing position to a kneeling position with no cushioning of the fall.

Pitcher. The base who directs the movement in the throw or toss of a toe pitch stunt.

Pony Sit. A partner stunt in which the base bends over with hands braced on the knees and the back flat. The top jumps up and sits on the base's back with legs tucked back.

Pyramid. A formation in which at least one person is supported off the ground by a base of two or more persons who are on the ground.

Roll-Down. A dismount from a partner stunt in which the top mount slowly rotates forward while maintaining contact with the base.

Roll-Off. A dismount from a shoulder sit in which the supporting surface for turning involves bodily contact with another person and is concluded with the feet landing on the ground.

Round-Off. A fast cartwheel with a half twist of the body so that a person lands on both feet simultaneously, and facing in the opposite direction.

Sailor T or Side T Lift. A partner stunt initiated from a standing side by side position. The base bends to the side to grasp the thigh and underarms of the top who jumps at a 45 degree angle over the base's shoulders. The base presses up to a locked arm position holding the top in a tight horizontal position.

Split. The act of lowering oneself to the floor with legs extended at right angles to the trunk.

Split Catch. A partner stunt in which the top is held in a tight spread eagle position (legs split apart, arms outstretched). The base's arms are locked overhead and support the top on the inside of each thigh.

Spotter. A person who assists in the building or dismounting of stunts and pyramids, watches for safety hazards (such as instability), and acts to prevent injuries. Spotters should always be in position with hands up and eyes on top mount.

Stunt. A formation which involves one person supporting another person off the ground.

Tension Drop. A stunt or pyramid in which all persons simultaneously lean forward in formation until the people on the top level jump forward off the base onto the ground. A tension drop is generally followed by a forward roll (sometimes referred to as a tension roll).

Twist. Rotation along the axis of the body.

Walkover. Slowly kicking the legs (one leg and then the other) over a handstand position in a forward or backward direction to land in an upright standing position.

Mounting Height Defined

A. ½ = Lunges (thigh stands), leg wraps, table tops (bent at waist), and, when sitting on shoulders, the distance between the shoulders of the bottom person and the shoulders of the top person.

B. 1 = One standing body height or standing with arms extended overhead.

C. 1½ = One standing body height as stated in B above **and** one of the halves as stated in A above.

D. 2 = Two standing body heights as stated in B above or one standing body height as stated in B above and two of the halves as stated in A above.

NOTE: These definitions are intended to assist in interpretation but cannot be all-inclusive for every situation. Concern for safety, awareness of current conditions, and common sense should be determining factors.

Joseph L. DeWalt

Heat-Related Illness

This chapter examines the clinical problems commonly encountered when people work or exercise in a hot, humid environment. Athletes are particularly susceptible to heat-related illnesses because of the relative intensity of their activities. Excessive heat buildup can do tremendous damage to the human body and, in extreme cases, may prove fatal. Taking the necessary precautions and exercising common sense can minimize the risk of heat-related illnesses.

The human body maintains a uniform core temperature of 98.6°F. Core temperature normally rises to between 101° and 103° within thirty minutes of commencing exercise, and this increase does not seriously impair body function. But if the core temperature rises to 106° to 108°, central nervous system functions deteriorate. Temperatures above 108°F can be fatal. Rectal temperature is a good measurement of core temperature.

Temperature Regulation

Heat is produced in the central core of the body as a byproduct of the metabolic processes that allow an athlete to compete. The circulatory system conducts this heat to the core's outer layer, the skin, where the body has several ways of dissipating the heat. Two of the most important ways are radiation and evaporation. When the temperature is 70°F or less, the body releases its heat into the environment by radiation. As

environmental temperatures approach the body's core temperature, however, heat loss through radiation is significantly reduced. In fact, athletes who practice in the hot August and September sun actually **gain** heat through radiation, and evaporation (sweating) is the only mechanism for effectively controlling core temperature. High temperatures and humidity do not compromise the performance of a well-hydrated, well-acclimatized athlete. But as exercise continues, water loss through sweating begins to inhibit the body's ability to cool itself. Exercise can be dangerous when environmental temperatures reach 105° or higher.

Sweat Glands

Studies have shown that the number of functional sweat glands an adult has is directly related to his or her environment. Adult men have more functioning sweat glands than adult women. When a person is subjected to physical stress that induces continual sweating, as time goes by the rate of sweating decreases and rectal temperature rises. This reduction in sweating is due to a decrease in the net flow per sweat gland and, to a lesser extent, to a decrease in the number of functioning sweat glands. Once sweat production begins to fall off, it does so sharply, and rectal temperature rises rapidly. This is due to swelling in one layer of the skin that mechanically blocks the opening of the sweat duct. The swelling is caused by absorption of sweat from the sur-

143

face of the skin and **can be prevented by drying the skin frequently during active sweating**. Acclimatization is a key factor, because previous exposure to heat determines how the sweat glands will respond.

Heat Illness Syndromes

• **Heat fatigue** is very common: 30 percent of athletes in outdoor sports experience it. Symptoms include weakness, tiredness, and lightheadedness. This mild condition is a warning to decrease or stop exercise and increase water consumption.

• **Heat syncope** (fainting) usually occurs at the end of a workout, such as the end of a race, when an athlete stops exercising abruptly and stands still. The athlete feels lightheaded and may actually faint (pass out). Lying down in a cool, shaded place, elevating the legs, and drinking water should alleviate the condition.

• **Heat cramps** are painful contractions that usually involve muscles of the lower extremities or the front of the abdomen. Cramps occur after intense, prolonged exercise and result from water loss and loss of body minerals such as salt, potassium, and calcium. Poorly acclimatized athletes are more susceptible, but any athlete who fails to maintain a diet that will replace salt and other minerals lost through exercise is at risk. Loss of calcium is especially significant for black athletes, because many blacks have a relative deficiency in the enzyme necessary to properly digest milk and dairy products, the principal suppliers of calcium. People with this enzyme deficiency have low levels of calcium even before exercise. However, they can easily circumvent the problem by supplementing their diets with calcium carbonate tablets (Tums).

Related to heat cramps is a syndrome commonly encountered on athletic playing fields but not described in medical texts. Coaches refer to this as **dead leg syndrome**. Dead leg syndrome typically appears after three to four weeks of intensive exercise in a hot, humid environment; the symptoms are extreme fatigue, weakness, and great difficulty in running. This syndrome is related to the inadequate replacement of potassium lost by sweating and can be prevented by supplementing the diet of the participating athlete with foods rich in potassium, particularly citrus fruits, bananas, or raisins.

• **Heat exhaustion** is a more serious, acute heat injury characterized by prostration, inability to concentrate, lightheadedness, hyperventilation, and lassitude. People with this condition sweat profusely and have a rapid pulse and a rectal temperature of 102° to 103°F. Heat exhaustion is caused by inadequate replacement of the water lost through sweat at the time of doing work. It can be prevented by allowing athletes to replace water adequately during activity. Weight charts that record an athlete's weight before and after practice are also helpful. Heat exhaustion is extremely unusual as long as weight loss during practices is kept to within 3 to 5 percent of total body weight.

An athlete with symptoms of heat exhaustion should be moved to a cool place and given plenty of cold water. Elevated temperature and decreased blood pressure are usual. If fluids taken orally do not relieve the symptoms, it may be necessary to give intravenous fluids. Keep an eye on any athlete who has required intravenous fluids for heat exhaustion after he or she returns to practice.

• **Heat stroke** is a medical catastrophe characterized by three major symptoms: rectal temperature of 106° or higher, marked mental confusion or unconsciousness (usually a coma), and shock. The best way to diagnose heat stroke is by rectal temperature. Because circulatory collapse is a major feature of heat stroke, it is not unusual for someone with this condition to have an oral temperature of 97° and a rectal temperature of 112°. The mortality (death) rate from heat stroke is directly related to the length and degree of temperature elevation. If the victim's temperature can be brought down to normal within 45 minutes of its first rise, the risk of death generally does not exceed 10 percent. When the temperature remains elevated for two hours, however, the mortality rate rises to 70 percent. Because time is such a crucial factor, coaches should immediately take athletes with symptoms of heat stroke to the nearest emergency room.

Heat stroke is more likely to occur in individuals who are poorly acclimatized, are obese, or consume alcohol. There is also evidence to indicate that the tendency toward heat stroke is inherited. Preparticipation physical exams should always include a question about any family history of heat illness.

Prevention

• **Acclimatization** (adjusting to heat) is defined as physiological changes that occur when the body is exposed to heat and that allow for more efficient heat regulation. A 4- to 8-day program of progressively longer periods of exercise in the heat improves the circulatory and sweating responses that dissipate heat, thus minimizing the incidence of heat exhaustion. The first day of the program should consist of exercise in light clothing for approximately 60 minutes. On each succeeding day, add 10 to 20 minutes and gradually increase the intensity of the exercise. If the sport is one requiring a uniform, the athletes should slowly change their clothing from shorts to partial uniform to full uniform. Eighty percent of acclimatization takes place within 7 days; it takes another 21 days for complete adjustment. Keep in mind that these figures are averages, and not all athletes will respond in the same way. Younger athletes, poorly conditioned athletes, and overweight athletes take longer to acclimatize. Identify these high-risk athletes early and have them watched closely for signs of heat illness.

• **Clothing**. Unless a sufficient amount of body surface area is exposed, sweat cannot evaporate and the body will not cool. For this reason, loose-fitting, white clothing is ideal for exercising in the heat. Football uniforms, by contrast, cover 50 percent of the skin's evaporation surfaces. Because 20 percent of the body's heat is lost through the head alone, evaporation can be enhanced by periodically removing helmets and exposing abdomens and legs as much as possible during break periods.

• **Water and salt replacement**. To minimize the risk of heat-related illnesses, **athletes should have unrestricted access to water during practices**. Two or three water breaks every hour are better than just one break an hour. Coaches and trainers should have water stations conveniently located at several places on the practice field and encourage water consumption.

Salt can be replaced by normal use of the salt shaker with meals. **Salt tablets are not recommended**. They just sit in the stomach and can cause more harm than good. Certain foods such as salted snack foods (e.g., potato chips), ham, and pizza are high in salt. Potassium lost through sweating can be replaced by following a diet rich in fruit and vegetables. Some good sources of calcium, which is important in the prevention and treatment of heat cramps, are milk, milk products, and cheese. Athletes who have difficulty digesting milk products can use calcium tablets (Tums) instead.

• **Drinks should be hypotonic (very little or no salt), cold, and low in sugar, and they should be consumed in amounts of three to ten ounces**. "Sports" drinks like Gatorade, Quick-Kick, or Pripps should be diluted with water (three parts water to one part drink). **The ideal drink is plain water**. Sports drinks are safe before or after games, but during competition they can actually prove harmful because they suppress thirst mechanisms, causing athletes to not drink enough to prevent dehydration.

• **Temperature and humidity**. The greater the humidity, the more difficult it is for the body to cool itself. A sling psychrometer measures wet bulb temperature, which provides a better gauge than regular temperature for estimating the potential danger of heat illness because it takes into account both temperature and humidity. Always measure the wet bulb temperature before a practice and adjust the intensity and duration of the practice session accordingly. Whenever the wet bulb temperature is under 60°F, no special precautions need be taken. If the wet bulb temperature is 61° to 65°, observe the players carefully. Whenever the wet bulb temperature is 71° to 75°, practice sessions should be shorter and rest breaks more frequent. A wet bulb temperature in excess of 75° indicates the need for extreme caution.

• **Weight charts**. The thirst mechanism does not always function well enough to ensure that an athlete replaces all the water lost with exercise. Keeping track of an athlete's body weight (in dry shorts) before and after practice can be helpful in making sure that weight lost during exercise has been regained by the following day. A postexercise weight loss of 2 to 3 percent of the total body weight is within normal range. Performance decreases when the weight loss exceeds 3 percent, and a total loss of 5 percent or more is a danger signal.

Implications

Before 1972 about five deaths a year were directly attributable to heat illness. Most of these deaths occurred during the first weeks of the practice season; the players were in full uniform and the temperature and humidity were at their maximum. Many of these casualties had not been allowed to drink water during practice and were required to take salt tablets. One fifteen-year-old athlete was garbed in a rubber suit in addition to his uniform and instructed to run laps. Rule changes in football have improved these statistics, **but there**

Heat-Related Illness **145**

are still too many deaths or near-deaths because coaches, trainers, and athletes do not understand how deadly heat can be. Although heat-related illness is most common in football, it can be a factor in any sport, especially spring sports because of warm weather late in the season. Coaches and trainers involved in all sports should know the symptoms of heat illness and should enforce preventative measures such as adequate hydration and acclimatization. Awareness can save lives.

Skin Problems
in Athletes

Skin problems are common in athletics because of increased body heat, perspiration, and friction from athletic gear. Contagious skin disorders are easily transmitted among athletes because of the close physical contact inherent to most sports. Meticulous attention to hygiene can help control most skin conditions, but the following problems can still prove troublesome, and some can lead to lost playing time.

Acne

Acne is a glandular skin disorder in which blockage of pores and the subsequent inflammation produces pimples, whiteheads, and blackheads. Acne abounds during the teen years; it is more severe in males than in females and is less common among Asians and blacks than among whites. An athlete's neck, upper arms, and trunk are the sites most often afflicted with acne.

Acne is made worse by excessive heat, humidity, mechanical irritation, touching or rubbing with the hands, stress, and cosmetics that don't allow the skin to breathe. The best treatment consists of washing with soap and water two to three times daily. Therapy should be aimed at reducing the amount of oil under the skin rather than the oil on the skin. Alcohol and other drying agents are generally ineffective. An athlete can apply benzoyl peroxide (oxy preparations) twice a day to reduce oil and unplug pores. An athlete with severe acne should see a physician. Antibiotics applied

to the skin or taken orally may help reduce the inflammation that goes along with acne.

Bacterial Infections

• **Impetigo**. **Staph** and **strep** bacteria cause the skin to become infected. The resulting lesions usually appear as scattered but discrete crusted sores the size of a dime. Sometimes these lesions become deep ulcers. Any skin lesion lasting more than three days is considered impetigo. Impetigo is treated with soap and water and oral antibiotics; topical antibiotics are usually not enough. **Keep in mind that impetigo is contagious**. Epidemics can occur in such close contact sports as wrestling. Early recognition is the key to preventing such outbreaks, so don't hesitate to have your team physician see any athlete who might have impetigo.

• **Boils**. A boil is a deep infection that develops in and around hair follicles. Boils begin as tender, hard, red bumps and then develop into larger, softer bumps filled with pus. Warm compresses applied for 20 minutes three times a day are sometimes sufficient treatment. Multiple boils require treatment with oral antibiotics such as penicillin. Boils may also need to be incised and drained by a physician. Because boils are contagious, athletes with draining boils should refrain from participation—particularly in contact or water sports—until treatment by a physician has begun.

147

Fungus Infections

• **Athlete's foot**. About 30 to 40 percent of all athletes experience the itching and macerated scaly rash between the toes and (occasionally) along the sides of the feet that comprise the symptoms of athlete's foot. Nonprescription drugs such as Tinactin and Micatin spray and cream usually cure the problem. If they don't, refer the athlete to a physician.

Athlete's foot can be **prevented** by: (1) wearing sandals or "flip-flops" in the shower; (2) washing feet thoroughly between toes and drying well; (3) treating any signs of athlete's foot early; (4) changing socks frequently.

• **Jock itch**. The characteristics of jock itch are severe itching and burning in the groin and a scaling rash in the area of the groin and buttocks. The rash typically appears as a raised ring surrounding a normal patch of skin. Ordinarily the scrotum is not involved.

Applying topical lotions such as Tinactin and Micatin three times a day for a week usually alleviates the condition. Do not use the spray forms of these medications, as they are very irritating. Caution male athletes against putting medication on the scrotum, which can also cause irritation. **Keep in mind that jock itch and athlete's foot frequently occur together**.

Viruses

• **Herpes (Type 1)**. The herpes simplex virus most commonly appears as a skin infection on the lips (fever blister) but can appear anywhere on the face, shoulders, and legs. Before the rash—which consists of clusters of blisters on a red base—appears, there may be burning and numbness present over the area of skin that will develop the rash. The blisters eventually rupture and crusts form. Healing can take between 10 and 21 days. Herpes can be recurrent.

Topical antibiotics such as Bacitracin can provide some relief from herpes sores. A drug exists that is effective against herpes if used very early, but it is expensive and must be prescribed by a physician. If an athlete suffers from recurring episodes of herpes, the physician may use this drug, which can be given orally or used topically.

• **Warts**. A wart is a tumor caused by a virus that most commonly appears on the hands, fingers, knees, or feet. Warts can be flat but usually are raised, hard,

ugly lesions. They eventually disappear on their own, but most people find them unsightly and want them removed immediately.

Physicians treat warts with salicylic acid plasters, liquid nitrogen, freezing, and various medications. They try to avoid surgery because it can result in a very painful scar, especially in the case of foot warts. Sometimes doughnut-shaped padding can provide temporary relief.

Lacerations

Stop the bleeding by applying pressure with a sterile gauze pad. Cleanse the wound with soap and water once the bleeding has stopped. If stitches appear necessary (either to stop the bleeding or because the wound is too large to be covered by "steri-strips"), apply a sterile compress and refer the athlete to a physician. Stitches need not be put in place immediately, but the delay should not exceed three or four hours. Find out when the athlete received his or her last tetanus shot. If it has been more than five years ago, the athlete should receive a booster.

Wounds always heal better if the edges are approximated with "steri-strips"; have the team physician demonstrate the use of these products. Keep the wound clean by changing the dressing daily and cleansing with hydrogen peroxide each time. Most athletes will be able to return to action the following day as long as the wound is protected with appropriate padding.

Abrasions

Abrasions, also known as strawberries or floor burns, should be cleansed with soap and water. Use a toothbrush to remove any dirt embedded in the abrasion and medicated ice to numb it. (For the latter, the team physician should provide lidocaine-novocaine. Combine this liquid with water in equal parts, freeze the solution, and apply the ice directly to the strawberry or floor burn for pain relief.)

Keep these scrapes as clean as possible with peroxide and apply antibiotic ointments to them. Superimposed infection is almost always preventable as long as the wound has been adequately cleaned. Watch for signs of infection (pain, heat, swelling, redness, and pus) and refer the athlete to the team physician if necessary. Do not overlook the possible need for a tetanus booster.

Blisters

Repeated rubbing against a localized area of skin can cause the accumulation of fluid in a sac called a blister. Blisters most commonly form over joints, the ends of fingers and toes, and the heel of the foot. Athletes may be alerted to a developing blister by a "hot spot," a reddened area under a poorly fitted shoe or piece of equipment. Use a sterile needle or lancet to drain blisters in several places, but keep the roof of the blister intact to promote faster healing. Cover a blister with antibiotic ointment and a dressing such as a Band-Aid or adhesive tape.

Athletes can prevent blisters by: (1) applying petroleum jelly to areas that rub, for example, the thighs and nipples of runners; (2) covering the sites of recurrent blisters with moleskin; (3) toughening skin by applying tincture of benzoin or soaking in tannic acid (strong tea) once a day for three weeks; (4) wearing new shoes several times before using them in practice or a game; (5) wearing two pairs of powdered socks, a thick pair under a thin pair; and (6) rubbing the pressure points of feet with a bar of soap before putting on socks. Perspiration will cause the soap to lather and reduce friction.

Sun-Damaged Skin

Many athletes relish the healthy and youthful appearance a suntan provides. However, nothing ages or damages the skin faster than exposure to sun. Encourage athletes who love to be in the sun to use sunscreens designed to effectively block the sun's harmful ultraviolet B (UVB) rays. Sunscreens are rated according to their ability to screen out UVB rays, which peak between the hours of 10:00 A.M. and 3:00 P.M. Low-grade sunscreens with a sun protection factor (SPF) of 5 allow some tanning with moderate protection against sunburn. Sunscreens with an SPF of 15 or higher provide more protection.

Treatment for sunburn consists of cooling the skin, preferably in a tub of cool water. Use ice compresses on blistered areas and anti-inflammatory drugs for pain relief.

Photosensitivity

Severe reddening of the skin on the face, arms, and legs (the most exposed areas of the body) after only a short exposure to the sun is known as **photosensitivity**. Photosensitivity can be caused by a medication the athlete is taking or by a substance applied to the skin. Deodorant soaps, perfumes (especially musk scent), and the antibiotic tetracycline are some of the more common causes. An athlete should treat photosensitivity by using sunscreens or by staying out of the sun when using one of the above-named irritants.

Dry Skin

This skin disorder worsens with exposure to dry weather or dry air. Bathing also aggravates the condition, because water and soap draw oil from the skin, causing "dishpan body." Athletes who shower several times a day often suffer from dry skin.

Symptoms include moderate itching of the legs with dry, scaling skin. The itching frequently ceases when the person is in the shower, only to recur 15 to 30 minutes afterward when the skin dries out. Swimmers often erroneously attribute their dry skin to chlorine.

Treatment consists simply of reducing the frequency of bathing. Athletes should limit their showers to two minutes or less after workouts and use such mild soaps as Dove or Ivory instead of deodorant bath soaps. They should also apply lubrication to their skin immediately after bathing and twice more daily. The ideal lubricant is petrolatum or Vaseline; however, many people find these substances objectionable. Such oils as mineral, bath, or baby oils are generally more acceptable.

Corns and Callouses

Callouses and corns consist of thickened skin over pressure points. Callouses are not tender; they are thickened areas that show skin markings and grooves on the surface and develop from chronic forces too weak to cause blisters. Callouses need not be treated but can be pared down by a health care provider if they become too large.

Corns are tender, compacted areas of skin that result from the compression of the skin between two unyielding surfaces (for example, between shoe and bone). Paring down a corn with a sharp knife or scalpel reveals a yellowish "kernel," and removal of this kernel relieves pain. Repeated paring or the use of corn plasters may help with persistent corns. Better-fitting shoes or shoe inserts may be necessary for recurring or difficult cases.

Anthony J. Geraci, Jr.

Common Medical Problems in Athletes

Such medical conditions as asthma, diabetes, seizure disorders, and hypertension are fairly common among high school athletes. In the past, these problems have been reason for excluding players from high school and college athletics, but we now know that people with underlying chronic medical conditions can safely participate in organized and individual sports and may actually benefit from the activity. Such participation is safest under the supervision of a physician who has been familiar with the individual case for some time and knows the effects of the disease on the particular athlete. Coaches, trainers, and team physicians should maintain close contact with this personal physician, especially when they are deciding on the athlete's suitability for participation.

People with medical problems can profit from athletics in ways beyond the usual benefits of exercise. In many cases, regular exercise can actually alter the effects of the condition; for example, it can improve lung function in asthmatics. Athletic participation also bolsters a person's self-esteem. This latter benefit is particularly important to young people for whom "fitting in" is an important factor in their personal happiness and sense of self-worth. Those responsible for de-

termining who will and who will not participate in athletic activities should strive to include anybody whose primary-care physician agrees, and physicians have a corresponding duty to suggest exercise and athletics to any of their patients who are able to take part.

This chapter examines several chronic medical disorders, the most common methods of treating each, and the side effects and benefits that can be expected from exercise.

Asthma

Asthma is a disease in which the lungs' air passages overreact to stimuli by constricting and making breathing difficult. Asthma often causes a high-pitched, breathy sound known as a wheeze. A number of stimuli can instigate an asthmatic response, depending on the individual. Some of the more common ones include dust, smoke, cold temperatures, exercise, and changes in the weather. One of these factors or a combination of them may trigger an attack; an asthmatic may also experience an attack for no apparent reason.

There are many treatments for asthma, including pills, syrups, and aerosolized sprays. Adjustments in the dosages of these drugs may be necessary as an asthmatic person progresses through an athletic training program. Asthmatics who complain of shortness of breath during exercise may be suffering an attack. They may need to use a prescribed inhalant to abort the attack and should be allowed to stop all activity until the episode has passed.

Emergency evaluation and treatment of an asthma attack is usually straightforward. **Symptoms** include fast breathing, shortness of breath, wheezing, and difficulty completing a sentence in one breath. **Treatment** may require only a couple of puffs of spray and rest. If able to speak, many asthmatics may be able to say what they need. Most asthma attacks that occur during exercise resolve within minutes. However, if no spray is nearby or if an attack continues even after use of the spray, the safest course is to call an ambulance for specialized treatment. Most ambulance personnel are trained to handle such cases should it be necessary. Some points to remember:

- If an athlete is asthmatic, ask his or her parents to provide a spare inhaler for the season. Keep this spray in the trainer's bag during practices and games in case an attack occurs. If there is more than one asthmatic on the team, label each athlete's spray. **Never let one athlete use another's medicine**.
- Aspirin and other medications such as ibuprofen (Advil, Nuprin, or Motrin) can trigger asthma attacks. An athlete whose asthma becomes worse may have taken one of these medications. Tylenol does not trigger asthma attacks and is therefore a safer pain reliever for muscular aches.
- Repeated episodes of coughing can be a symptom of asthma. Athletes who cough during or immediately after exercise may have asthma and need to be evaluated by a physician.
- Exercise-induced asthma can be prevented with a spray given 30 minutes before exercise.
- Remember that there are many outstanding athletes who have asthma.

Diabetes

Diabetes (diabetes mellitus, "sugar") occurs in 3 percent of the population. There are two types of diabetes, one requiring daily insulin injections and one not requiring insulin, but both have in common a deficiency of the actions of the hormone insulin, which controls sugar metabolism within the body. Only the insulin-dependent type is discussed here, because almost all adolescent diabetics need insulin.

The most common problem for diabetics during exercise is low blood sugar. Although high blood sugar can also occur, it is much harder to diagnose, and the emergency treatment is the same as for low blood sugar. **Symptoms** in the early stages of low blood sugar include tremulousness (athlete appears nervous or shaky), hunger, headache, or lightheadedness. Diabetics frequently know when their sugar level is getting low. Sometimes a diabetic with sugar abnormalities may seem confused, sweaty, or tired. If this happens, and the athlete is alert enough to swallow, putting granulated sugar or frosting under the tongue may help. If the diabetic is unconscious or is not alert enough to swallow, **nothing** should be put in the mouth. Diabetics suffering from such reactions may even look **and smell** drunk; any diabetic who seems intoxicated should be presumed to be suffering from an insulin reaction. In any of these circumstances, you should call an ambulance if the athlete does not improve immediately.

If diabetics begin to feel the symptoms indicating that their blood sugar is out of control, they may need to eat a sugar-laden snack immediately and should be allowed to have some fruit juice or other sugar-containing liquid or a piece of hard candy. In a pinch, any food containing sugar helps. **Whenever diabetics state that they need to eat, they should be allowed to do so**, as this usually forestalls serious problems later. It would be prudent to keep some hard candy or sugar packets in the team first-aid kit whenever a diabetic athlete participates in organized sports. Diabetics are also particularly sensitive to dehydration, and adequate fluids should be readily available.

The **treatment** of diabetes includes insulin injections, special diets, and regular adjustment of the insulin dosage based on activity level. Diabetics must be in close contact with their personal physicians during the early stages of training. In most circumstances, the team physician should defer to the judgment of the diabetic's personal physician regarding changes in treatment because of exercise. Most diabetics actually gain increased sugar control with exercise and should be encouraged to participate in athletics. Close communication among athlete, trainer, coaches, and primary-care physician is an important factor in allaying any apprehension that might arise from participation.

Seizure Disorders (Epilepsy), Convulsions

Epilepsy is a very mysterious and frightening condition to those who do not understand it. It takes many forms, from simple staring spells or spells of inattentiveness to generalized contractions of all the muscles in the body. All these manifestations are caused by the uncoordinated firing of certain nerves in the brain, and most can be controlled by medications that decrease such nerve activity. Only the prospective athlete's primary-care physician can state whether a certain sport is safe for the patient, and under what circumstances. Most people with seizure disorders can participate in all sports.

Once the physician approves an athlete's participation, there is rarely any need to alter regular training methods. Athletes with seizure disorders can attain the same level of fitness and excellence as those without a history of seizures.

A person with a seizure disorder can have an attack at any time. For this reason, it is important for coaches to know what form the seizures are likely to take in a particular athlete, so that they will recognize an episode when it occurs. In the event of a seizure, **the first priority is to prevent injury**. The person should be held gently to prevent him or her from striking hard objects with flailing limbs, and all equipment should be moved out of reach. **Never place anything in the mouth of someone who is having a seizure!** One frequent response is to place a spoon in the person's mouth to prevent tongue biting. Experience has shown, however, that the complications of damaged teeth and swallowed spoons are far more dangerous than any potential injury to the tongue.

Knowing how to give first aid for seizures is an important skill for coaches and trainers, because many seizures occur in individuals who have never had one before. Training programs and situations that predispose an athlete to dehydration and hypothermia (e.g., marathons) also lower the brain's seizure threshold. During a seizure, place the athlete on one side rather than on the back or face down. This position facilitates proper breathing and allows any spit or vomit to drain from the mouth. Remain calm; seizures stop in one or two minutes, although it may seem longer. Once the seizure stops, the athlete may be unresponsive for a few minutes. Respiration will be shallow; feel the athlete's pulse

to reassure yourself that he or she is not suffering cardiac arrest. After five to ten minutes the athlete usually rouses but may be dazed, confused, and weak. People often feel embarrassed after a seizure. Be sensitive to their feelings; an empathetic approach at the time of seizure may prevent an athlete's withdrawal from athletics due to embarrassment.

A **convulsion** (seizure) can also be a sign of head injury, so knowledge of the events preceding the seizure is important. If an athlete has just been involved in a collision or has been having headaches following an earlier collision, a serious head injury must be considered (see Chapter 7, "Head and Neck Injuries"). Emergency room evaluation is essential when a seizure occurs after a head injury. **All athletes who have had a seizure should see a physician to obtain medical clearance before playing again**.

High Blood Pressure

High blood pressure in a young athlete is usually discovered through a high school sports physical. Young men, especially blacks, have a higher incidence of high blood pressure. Exercise is an excellent treatment for high blood pressure principally because it contributes to weight reduction and decreased tension.

Any athlete with a big arm will have a "false" high blood pressure reading unless a large blood pressure cuff is used. Weight lifting can also elevate blood pressure. Certain medications—for example, diuretics or beta blockers—that are sometimes used to treat hypertension can cause problems such as dehydration and reduced capacity for an athlete during exercise. All hypertensive athletes should be fully evaluated by their primary-care physicians before they participate in any sport.

Mononucleosis

Infectious mononucleosis, or "mono," occurs most frequently in teenagers and young adults. It is caused by a virus and is usually a mild illness that lasts from one to three weeks. Tiredness, low-grade fever, swollen lymph nodes, and a sore throat are the most common symptoms.

Mononucleosis is not a very contagious disease, so isolating a player from his or her teammates is not necessary. Fatigue is a common trait of this illness, but its severity varies from person to person. Treat each athlete individually. A person with mono should be allowed to participate as long as his or her performance is closely monitored. Let demonstrated endurance be your guide.

If the athlete is involved in a contact sport like football, basketball, or soccer, a more thorough examination is warranted. Mononucleosis usually causes the spleen to become enlarged, which increases its chances of rupturing. It is generally not advisable to allow an athlete with an enlarged spleen to participate in contact sports.

Other Conditions

There are many other chronic and acute medical conditions that may be found in people who wish to participate in athletics. In most cases, exercise is not only permissible but beneficial. Close cooperation among athlete, trainer, coaches, and physicians assures the safest and fullest participation possible. Rigid rules, such as the one (common twenty years ago) forbidding participation in high school athletics by any person with a heart murmur, benefit neither the athlete nor the sport. No matter what the health problem, there probably is some sport that will prove salutary.

Some chronic medical problems require the use of medications. Needles and pills have a negative image in today's society, and any athlete seen using them will certainly be stigmatized. It is important for you to know what medications your athletes use and to ask for a physician's note authorizing the use of these medications and explaining any side effects.

Playing with Fever

Many illnesses—even a simple viral infection—can cause a fever. It is probably a good rule of thumb to keep an athlete from participating while he or she has a fever unless cleared by a physician. This is the safest practice because a fever may cause difficulties in regulating body temperature.

Salli Benedict

24

Nutritional Concerns for the Athlete

The Basics of Good Nutrition

The basics of good nutrition for high school athletes are simple: The right diet consists of a normal, healthy diet with the addition of extra calories to cover growth, development, and added physical activity. An athlete's diet may also need to include extra iron, because iron deficiency is common among teenage girls. Athletes should eat such iron-rich foods as eggs, iron-fortified cereals, whole grains, dried beans, and nuts. An inadequate supply of iron creates a condition called **anemia**, which can interfere with normal growth; symptoms of a deficiency include lack of energy, fatigue, and increased susceptibility to infection. Consult a physician if an athlete shows symptoms of anemia.

In a healthy diet, 15 percent of the total calories come from protein sources, 30 percent or less from fats, and the remaining 55 percent from carbohydrates. Extra calories added to this normal diet should come from carbohydrates, which are also good sources of vitamins, minerals, and fiber. Protein is an expensive source of calories, and consumption of fats should be minimized in order to help prevent heart disease. Contrary to the myths that stress the importance of protein, most athletes **do not need to increase their protein intake beyond the normal level eaten by most teenagers**.

A healthy, well-balanced diet consists of daily choices from the basic four food groups:

- **Dairy products** (four servings)—low-fat or skim milk, cheese, yogurt, cottage cheese, ice cream, ice milk, frozen yogurt
- **Meat and protein** (three servings)—lean meats, chicken, fish, dried beans, tofu, nuts, eggs
- **Breads and cereals** (four or more servings)—breads (preferably whole grain, including muffins, bagels, pizza dough), cold and hot cereals (preferably iron fortified), pasta, rice
- **Fruits and vegetables** (four or more servings)—all fruits and vegetables, including citrus fruits and leafy green and bright orange vegetables daily

Teenagers are notorious for the amounts of fast food, sugars, and fats they consume. Skipping meals and snacking are routine. Because a teenage athlete is interested in improving performance, he or she may be more willing to listen to suggestions for good nutrition. Coaches, trainers, team physicians, and parents should take this opportunity to emphasize eating habits that can improve health and athletic performance. Teenagers do **not** have to forgo favorite "junk" foods like ice cream, hamburgers, pizza, and soft drinks, which can still play a part in their overall diet. Problems arise when **most** of their diet comes from these foods, which are high in fat and sugar and low in vitamins and minerals.

Most teenage athletes require a high caloric intake. The average sixteen-year-old girl consumes about 2,500 calories a day; boys consume about 3,500. Training and competition burn up an additional 500 to 1,500 calories. Boys involved in such endurance sports as cross-country running or cycling may need as many as 6,000 calories a day. Simply finding the time to eat that much food can be a problem, and frequent snacks as well as three large meals a day are necessary. An example of a high-calorie meal plan is shown in Table 1 under "Sample Meal Plans" below.

Water and Other Fluids

There are several nutritional concerns related to hydration that go beyond those covered in Chapter 21. An adequate fluid intake is crucial for all athletes, but teenage athletes are particularly susceptible to heat-related illnesses and therefore must be carefully monitored. A general guideline for ensuring proper hydration is to consume one quart of water for every 1,000 calories of food eaten. A teenager who consumes 5,000 calories a day needs five quarts of water or other acceptable fluids. Because thirst is a poor indicator of the quantity of fluids needed, **athletes should never wait until they are thirsty to drink**. They should begin practice or an event with a well-hydrated body and should replenish lost water throughout an event. Water is by far the best liquid to consume before and during an event. Diluted sports drinks such as Gatorade, Quick-Kick, or 10K are also acceptable; full-strength sports drinks have high sugar contents, which can slow down emptying of the liquid from the stomach and cause a feeling of fullness or even nausea and vomiting.

Some general guidelines for what athletes should drink include:

• **3 hours before event**—three or more glasses of water, low-fat milk, fruit juice, lemonade, diluted pineapple juice, clear broth, or bouillon
• **90 to 30 minutes before event**—two glasses of water, carbonated mineral water, sports drink, or diet cola

• **During event**—at least two glasses of cool water every hour (more in hot, humid weather)
• **After event**—water, carbonated mineral water, Gatorade, colas, fruit juices

The Pregame Meal

The purpose of a pregame meal is to give athletes the energy they need for competition, to keep them from getting hungry during an event without upsetting their stomachs, to make sure their bodies are well hydrated, and (perhaps most important) to give them a psychological boost. Athletes may be disappointed to learn that the traditional steak-and-potatoes pregame meal is **not** the best choice. The following guidelines for pregame meals may be helpful:

• Eat three hours before the game. This allows time for digestion but should prevent hunger. (Steak requires five to six hours for adequate digestion and does not provide any energy until the next day.)
• Try to make the meal enjoyable. Psychological factors have as much or more to do with performance as the actual content of the meal.
• Keep fat and protein at or below recommended levels. Too much fat slows digestion. Too much protein can prevent adequate hydration.
• Include plenty of carbohydrates for needed energy.
• Drink three or more glasses of fluid with the meal.
• Avoid very salty foods like potato chips, ham, cold cuts, and hot dogs, all of which cause thirst.
• Avoid such "gassy" foods as carbonated drinks and beans.
• A liquid pregame meal can be ideal for athletes who have "queasy" stomachs before competition. Sustagen, Sustacal, and Ensure are acceptable substitutes for a solid meal and have the advantage of being lactose free, an aid to the 60 percent of blacks and 90 percent of Asians who cannot tolerate milk.

Sample pregame meals are shown in Table 2.

Glycogen or Carbohydrate Loading

Glycogen or carbohydrate loading is a technique for greatly increasing the amount of glycogen stored in a muscle, which in turn directly affects the endurance of that muscle. In the first phase of the regimen, six and five days before the event, respectively, an athlete depletes stored glycogen by restricting carbohydrate intake and training intensely. In the second phase, days four, three, and two before the event, the athlete consumes large amounts of carbohydrates and minimizes fat and protein intake, while also cutting back on training. On the day of the event, the athlete maintains a normal diet consistent with pregame meal and hydration guidelines. This regimen has been shown to help endurance athletes. Nevertheless, because the first phase can cause extreme fatigue and may compromise academic performance, **it is strongly recommended that adolescents avoid the first phase of the glycogen loading regimen**. Instead, they should consume a normal diet during the first part of the week preceding a game or event, followed by a high-carbohydrate diet for a few days just before the event.

Weight Control for the Teenage Athlete

Maintaining the right balance between caloric intake and energy expenditure to ensure proper growth and physical development as well as optimal athletic performance can be a challenge to young athletes. For those who wish to gain or lose weight, there are additional medical and nutritional considerations.

Gaining Weight

Many athletes, but especially football players, weightlifters, shot-putters, and discus throwers, want to gain weight in order to improve their performance. The goal of weight gain is to increase **muscle** (lean body mass) rather than fat. Muscle mass can only be increased by combining muscle workouts with increased caloric intake. There are no special substances, including proteins or vitamins and drugs, that magically increase muscle mass. Although a relatively small amount of additional protein is needed for muscle development, the daily intake of virtually all teenagers is more than enough to meet this requirement. Therefore protein supplements are not recommended, as they may have undesirable side effects.

The recommended rate of weight gain is about one to two pounds per week, a rate that usually can be attained by adding between 500 and 1,000 calories per day to the diet. Faster weight gain usually indicates an increase in fat rather than muscle. Muscle training must be part of the weight-gain program; otherwise the extra calories will convert to fat. See Table 1 for a high-calorie meal pattern.

Losing Weight

Gymnasts, wrestlers, dancers, and long-distance runners are usually concerned with maintaining a low body weight. Some of the methods they use to lose weight are not conducive to peak athletic performance and furthermore may impede normal growth and development. Fasting, restricting fluids, self-induced vomiting, sitting in saunas, and taking laxatives, diuretics, and enemas should all be avoided. These methods usually cause a reduction in muscle strength and are associated with lowered blood volume, decreased oxygen consumption, depleted glycogen stores, and low blood sugar (hypoglycemia). Wrestlers probably run the greatest risks through rapid weight loss due to their pattern of dropping weight before a match and rapidly regaining it afterward, which not only increases their risk of dehydration but also breaks down muscle. Wrestlers should follow the same weight-loss program as other athletes. The minimum level of body fat is 5 to 7 percent for males and 10 percent for females, as determined by skin calipers. Adolescents should never fall below these levels. Weight loss should always be gradual (one to two pounds per week), because a faster loss results in decreased muscle mass. Any weight loss program should ensure an adequate intake of calories and nutrients to sustain growth and normal physical performance. Adolescents should not consume fewer than 1,800 to 2,200 calories per day. Instead, weight should be lost by reducing caloric intake by 500 to 700 calories per day and by increasing energy expenditure by 500 to 700 calories per day. Table 3 shows an 1,800-calorie and a 2,400-calorie meal plan. Whenever you work with an athlete in a weight-loss program, be sure to consult with the parents and team physicians and monitor the athlete's weight and body composition weekly.

Sample Meal Plans

Abbreviations:

c. = cup   oz. = ounce
tsp. = teaspoon   cal. = calories
Tbsp. = Tablespoon

Table 1. High-Calorie Sample Meal Plan
(approximately 6,000 calories)

Breakfast: ¾ c. orange juice; 1 c. hot cereal with 2 tsp. sugar; 1 egg, fried; 1 slice whole wheat toast with 1 tsp. margarine, 1 tsp. jelly; 8 oz. milk (whole).
Total cal. = 620

Snack: 1 peanut butter and jelly sandwich (2 slices bread, 2 Tbsp. peanut butter, 2 tsp. jelly); ½ c. raisins; 1 c. apple juice.
Total cal. = 680

Lunch: 1 ham and cheese sandwich (2 slices bread, 1 oz. cheese, 1 oz. ham, 1 Tbsp. mayonnaise); 1 serving french fries; 1 c. tossed green salad with 2 Tbsp. dressing; 10-oz. chocolate milkshake; 4 oatmeal cookies.
Total cal. = 1,440

Snack: 1 bagel with 2 tsp. margarine and 2 Tbsp. cream cheese; 1 c. sweetened applesauce; ¾ c. grape juice.
Total cal. = 710

Dinner: 2 pieces baked chicken (7 oz. total); 1 c. rice with 1 tsp. margarine; 1 c. collard greens; ½ c. candied sweet potatoes; 2 pieces cornbread with 1 Tbsp. margarine; 8 oz. milk (whole); 1 slice apple pie.
Total cal. = 1,760

Snack: 1 banana; ½ c. peanuts; 1 c. chocolate milk (whole).
Total cal. = 720

Table 2. Sample Pregame Meals
(to be eaten 3 to 4 hours prior to event)

• ¾ c. orange juice; ½ c. cereal with 1 tsp. sugar; 1 slice whole wheat toast with: 1 tsp. margarine and 1 tsp. honey or jelly; 8 oz. skim or low-fat milk; water.
Total cal. = 450–500

• ¾ c. orange juice; 1 to 2 pancakes with: 1 tsp. margarine and 2 Tbsp. syrup; 8 oz. skim or low-fat milk; water.
Total cal. = 450–500

• 1 c. vegetable soup; 1 turkey sandwich with 2 slices bread, 2 oz. turkey (white or dark), 1-oz. cheese slice, 2 tsp. mayonnaise; 8 oz. skim or low-fat milk; water.
Total cal. = 550–600

• 1 c. spaghetti with tomato sauce and cheese; ½ c. sliced pears (canned) on ¼ c. cottage cheese; 1 to 2 slices Italian bread with 1 to 2 tsp. margarine (avoid garlic); ½ c. sherbet; 1 to 2 sugar cookies; 4 oz. skim or low-fat milk; water.
Total cal. = 700

Table 3. Sample Meal Plans for Losing Weight

1,800 Calories:

Breakfast: ¾ c. orange juice; ¾ c. cereal; 8 oz. low-fat milk; 1 slice whole wheat toast with 1 tsp. margarine.
Total cal. = 415

Snack: 1 apple.
Total cal. = 80

Lunch: 1 peanut butter and banana sandwich (2 slices bread, 1 Tbsp. peanut butter, ½ banana); 5 to 7 carrot sticks; 1 peach; 8 oz. low-fat milk.
Total cal. = 485

Snack: 20 grapes; 2 graham crackers.
Total cal. = 155

Dinner: 1 hamburger patty (4 oz.) with 1 hamburger bun; 1 c. tossed green salad with 1 Tbsp. dressing; 4 oz. low-fat milk; ½ c. ice cream.
Total cal. = 715

2,400 Calories:

Breakfast: ¾ c. orange juice; 1 slice toast with 1 oz. cheese; ¾ c. cereal; 4 oz. low-fat milk.
Total cal. = 420

Snack: 1 banana.
Total cal. = 100

Lunch: 1 slice cheese pizza; 1 cup tossed green salad with 1 Tbsp. dressing; 8 oz. low-fat milk.
Total cal. = 425

Snack: ½ c. raisin/peanut mix; ½ c. apple juice.
Total cal. = 360

Dinner: 1 c. macaroni and cheese; ½ c. lima beans; 1 c. tomato and cucumber slices with 1 Tbsp. dressing; 1 dinner roll with 1 tsp. margarine; 8 oz. low-fat milk.
Total cal. = 895

Snack: ½ c. sherbet; 1 granola cookie.
Total cal. = 185

Table 4. High-Carbohydrate Sample Meal Plan

Breakfast: ¾ c. orange or pineapple juice; 1 egg, fried; 2 slices toast with 2 tsp. margarine and 2 tsp. jelly; ¾ c. cereal; 8 oz. skim or low-fat milk or hot cocoa.

Lunch: 1 or 2 sandwiches, each with 1 oz. meat or 1 oz. cheese or 2 Tbsp. peanut butter; carrot and celery sticks; 1 banana; 8 oz. skim or low-fat milk.

Dinner: 5 to 6 oz. baked fish or chicken without skin; 1 baked potato with 1 tsp. margarine; ½ c. green beans; ½ c. coleslaw; 2 pieces cornbread with 2 tsp. margarine and 2 tsp. honey; ½ c. sliced peaches; 8 oz. skim or low-fat milk.

Snacks: 1 or 2 servings of fruit; 1 or 2 servings of cookies/crackers.

Michael J. DeBevec

25

The Woman Athlete

The differences in athletic abilities between men and women are smaller than was once thought. Physicians have proved that many once-common beliefs are nothing but myths that have hindered the progress of women's athletics. Exposing these fallacies has led to the realization that women have enormous potential for improving their athletic performance. This chapter reviews some of the myths that continue to impede women's athletics and focuses on some of the unique problems faced by women athletes.

Body Fat

Women have, on average, 10 percent more body fat than men. As with men, the distribution of this fat is determined more by ethnic origin, hormonal status, and choice of sport than by any specific type of training. The total amount of body fat in a woman athlete varies with the sport—it is lowest in runners, gymnasts, and ballet dancers and highest in swimmers and basketball and volleyball players. Current studies indicate that one cannot lose weight selectively from certain areas of the body, contradicting a myth promulgated by the seller of many gimmicks and gadgets that promise to alter female body shape. Increased activity is the surest way to reduce total body fat.

Muscular Development

Muscular development is the area in which erroneous beliefs have most contributed to the inequality in athletic programs for women. The quality of muscle tissue is identical in both sexes. Women tend as a rule to have weaker upper bodies than men, but they have equal or greater potential for strength increases, with the average potential increase for a woman athlete being 15 to 45 percent. A woman's outward appearance does not change appreciably with strength training because her subcutaneous fat tends to hide the muscular definition or prominent veins associated with weight training. A woman's flexibility, motor coordination, and speed, just like a man's, do not diminish with increasing strength. Women can tolerate rigorous muscle training programs, both physically and psychologically, and should be encouraged to include such programs as part of their training for any sport that requires either endurance or explosive bursts of effort.

Bones

In comparison to men, women have lighter skeletons, narrower shoulders, and wider hips relative to the total body size, and they usually weigh thirty to forty pounds less for a given height. Bone density is generally less in adult women than in men. The biggest difference between the sexes is the size and shape of a woman's pelvis, which plays a vital role in childbearing. These skeletal differences contribute to the increased incidence of the following disorders in women: subluxations, dislocations, and pain in the kneecap; bursitis and bunions; stress fractures in the leg and hip; and bursitis of the hip. The incidence of knee sprains and ankle sprains is the same for both men and women. Female athletes who are not well conditioned have a higher incidence of overuse injuries.

Aerobic Function

A woman's aerobic function differs somewhat from a man's. The usual index of aerobic function is maximum oxygen uptake—the ability of the heart to pump blood and oxygen to the muscles, which thereby determines the amount of oxygen taken up by the muscles. Several factors have an effect on maximum oxygen uptake, including the size and pumping ability of the heart and the hemoglobin level in the blood. These factors are approximately 10 to 25 percent greater in men than women due to hormonal and genetic differences. However, female athletes have the ability to increase their maximum oxygen uptake as much as 30 percent. With training, many women can achieve a higher oxygen uptake than some men.

Heat Tolerance

Another myth contradicted by recent studies holds that women are less able to tolerate heat stress than men. There are differences in women that affect heat regulation, including a lower basal metabolic rate, a thicker layer of subcutaneous fat, and fewer functioning sweat glands. **However, well-conditioned women can tolerate exercise in the heat as well as men.**

Weight Loss

Female athletes interested in losing weight should first come to an agreement with their coaches and/or physicians about an ideal performance weight. This ideal weight can be calculated in the following manner:

• The basic weight for a woman five feet tall is 105 pounds.

• Add five pounds for every inch over five feet (e.g., a 5'4" woman would have an ideal weight of 125 pounds).

That ideal weight can vary as much as 15 percent in either direction without compromising the general health of the athlete. In certain sports, peak performance may be related to significant deviations from the norm. For instance, female runners perform better at a lower weight, whereas female swimmers may perform better at a higher weight.

The basic strategy for weight loss is to increase the duration of workouts while decreasing caloric intake and maintaining a well-balanced diet. An athlete should consume an adequate amount of food and should drink at least eight glasses of low-calorie fluids such as water per day. Restrictive weight-loss diets, such as a low protein diet, or use of dietary aids, diet pills, and the like are inadvisable.

Women athletes who want to gain weight should avoid anabolic steroids or high-protein diets. The best way to gain weight is to increase caloric intake in a well-balanced diet while simultaneously increasing specific strength training (see Chapter 24).

Anemia

About 20 to 30 percent of female athletes need to take iron supplements because of either poor dietary habits or excess loss of blood through menstruation. Some physicians and sports medicine advisers routinely recommend iron supplements for women. Any woman with inadequate iron intake or heavy menstrual periods should have routine blood tests to screen for iron-deficiency anemia.

The Breast

A variety of myths and misconceptions regarding the breast in relation to athletics need to be clarified. A female's breast is composed mostly of fat tissue rather than muscle. Exercise does not increase the size of a breast, although hypertrophy of the underlying pectoralis muscle, which would occur in a strength training program, can give the chest a certain fullness in appearance. No specific exercise decreases the breast's size either. Loss of weight may decrease general body fat stores, proportionally decreasing the size of the breast but, contrary to popular belief, localized fat loss from the breast is impossible.

The two major problems likely to affect an athlete's breasts during competition are soreness and contusions. The amount of soreness is directly related to the vertical (up and down) movement of the breasts during activity. A variety of **sports bras** on the market, designed to protect breasts during competition, work to prevent soreness by limiting vertical movement. Breasts are no more likely to receive trauma than any other part of the body and can be protected with inserts or pads in the bra. When purchasing bras, women should look for nonirritating seams, fasteners that will not rub against the torso, and nonslip straps. Bras that will be worn during sports that require overhead arm activity should have stretchy straps. Women who choose not to wear a bra sometimes develop "jogger's nipple," an irritation that results from the nipple's rubbing against the overlying garment. This condition can, of course, be treated by wearing a bra or by placing a large Band-Aid over the nipple during exercise. "Jogger's nipple" is more common in cold weather and also affects males.

Menstrual Periods

The onset of menstruation in adolescence is directly related to total weight and/or total body fat. A body fat total of 17 percent is required for the onset of menstruation and 22 percent to maintain normal menstrual function. It also appears that in most cases menstruation tends to begin when a girl's weight reaches around 100 pounds. The average menstrual period lasts between three and seven days; the flow is heavier at the beginning and lighter at the end. Menstruation normally occurs every twenty-one to twenty-six days.

A girl usually has her first menstrual period at about age twelve, but she might be anywhere from nine to sixteen. **In general, athletes tend to begin menstruation later**, which provides a certain selective competitive advantage in such sports as gymnastics. The delay is probably related to a delay in achieving a body fat percentage or absolute weight that would bring on menses, although training and stress have not been eliminated as causative agents. Delayed onset of menstrual periods does not influence later fertility, but there is some concern within the medical community that a

lack of menstrual periods may cause thin bones. Because of these concerns, an athlete who is not having periods by age fourteen or who has menstruated but then stops should be evaluated by a physician.

Lack of menstrual periods is a common occurrence in female athletes involved in any sport that involves regular endurance training or minimization of body weight or body fat percentage. One cannot assume, however, that absent menstrual periods in a woman athlete are necessarily due to her involvement in a sport or training. Such an assumption might cause one to overlook other disorders such as pregnancy or tumors. Also, there is a high incidence of anorexia nervosa among athletes without menstrual periods. **The following are signs that warrant physician referral**:

- No menstrual period by age fourteen
- Menstrual period does not return after the end of a period of heavy training or at the end of a competitive season
- Six months, or the equivalent of three menstrual cycles, without a menstrual period when the athlete has previously had normal periods
- Suspicion of anorexia nervosa based on such symptoms as binge eating and/or bouts of vomiting; athlete thinks she is overweight but is actually underweight
- Suspicion of possible pregnancy

Performance is not necessarily affected by menses alone, but it may be affected by premenstrual syndrome (PMS) and cramps. PMS usually begins three to four days before the period. The symptoms are increased irritability, weight gain, and decreased motivation. Menstrual cramps can be severe. The first few years that a young girl menstruates, she may not have cramps because she is not ovulating (making an egg), but once ovulation begins her periods may become painful. Both of these problems can be treated. Evaluation by a physician is recommended for any athlete who finds that cramps or PMS interferes with her athletic performance.

Women in contact sports run no greater risk of internal organ damage that could result in sterility than do men.

Conclusion

Recent studies indicate that women are capable of making great strides in athletic performance. In order to realize their athletic potential, however, women must take advantage of new information regarding participation in competitive athletics. Like men, they should choose a sport wisely, taking into consideration body type and other demonstrated or inherited skills. Strength training programs are particularly important for competitive women athletes. And women as well as men should participate in endurance training and in stretching programs that promote flexibility. Finally, women should not hesitate to seek appropriate professional guidance for any medical or training problems.

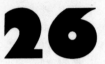

John C. LaLonde

Sports
Psychology

There has been an upsurge of interest in sports psychology over the past few years as coaches, trainers, and physicians have come to realize that despite improved coaching, better equipment, and changes in rules, athletes are suffering injuries as frequently as ever. This chapter examines the relationship between psychology and injuries in athletics as well as some emotional problems that adversely affect an athlete's health.

Emotion and Injury

Research indicates that various psychological factors, such as personality characteristics and emotional states, can contribute to an injury. Athletes who are hostile and aggressive, detached and reserved, or extremely critical of self or others seem to run a higher risk of injury. Emotional factors that can predispose an athlete to injury include family stress resulting from conflict or pressure within the home, social problems involving peers, or academic pressure. One study showed that if a parent has recently died, the athlete is five times more likely to suffer an injury.

Injury-prone Athletes

Psychological factors may also help explain the phenomenon of "injury-prone" athletes. Often these athletes are simply victims either of physical traits that make them more susceptible to injury or of just plain bad luck. However, injuries can also be a means of escape or revenge for athletes with psychological problems. Athletes who do not enjoy their sport or who have been pressured into participating by athletically frustrated parents or enthusiastic friends may find that injury is a socially acceptable way to escape the activity while simultaneously gaining sympathy. Athletes with low self-esteem may promote an injury as a sign of courage or may look on it as a form of self-punishment. **This is not to say that all injuries have a psychological cause or that you should automatically question the validity of an injury**. Try to be aware of circumstances affecting athletes' psychological health, but remember that athletes are often unaware of any psychological causes of their injuries. Athletes who have problems need help, not condemnation. If you suspect a psychological problem, have a private conversation with the athlete and try to find out if there is actually a problem. Don't be too pushy; give each athlete appropriate time and space to deal with the issue. He or she may come back another time and be ready to talk.

Psychological Problems Caused by Injuries

Injuries can also be the cause of psychological problems in athletes. The psychological consequences of an injury can be as varied as the factors that led to the injury. Athletes initially may try to deny that they are injured. They may not seek help, knowing that the trainer will force them to sit out until the injury heals. They may try to bargain with the trainer about the seriousness of an injury. This should never be a bargaining point, however, because untreated injuries leave athletes susceptible to further injury and possibly to permanent damage.

Injuries may also cause feelings of anger, blame, and depression. An athlete who perceives the injury as a disaster may be overwhelmed with anxiety and become irrational. Very often an athlete's entire identity and sense of self-worth revolves around the sport and his or her ability to perform. Anything that threatens the ability to participate appears to threaten the athlete's very existence. Coaches and trainers can help the athlete put the injury into perspective by portraying it as an opportunity to show courage. It is important to legitimize feelings of disbelief, frustration, anger, and so on while at the same time helping athletes to realize that their self-worth is not contingent upon athletic ability.

Keep in mind that injury evaluation can have important psychological implications. Athletes feel most vulnerable at the time they are injured. You should remain calm and in control regardless of the circumstances. Choose your words carefully; an athlete hears not only what is said, but what is not said. It is vitally important that injured athletes feel that the person treating them has their best interests in mind.

Rehabilitation and Psychology

Psychology also plays an important role in rehabilitation. You should always be supportive and make injured athletes feel that they are still part of the team. Inform them of the "whys and hows" of rehabilitation—the better informed they are, the more compliant they will be. Provide a timetable indicating the goals to be reached and how to reach them, and give super-vision when needed. Some athletes need constant supervision to prevent their doing too much or too little; others need little or none. Give feedback on the athlete's progress. Above all, use positive reinforcement. Most athletes already have enough negative feelings to last a lifetime; you don't need to add to them.

Preventing Injuries

An awareness of psychological factors that can predispose someone to injury can aid in prevention. Keep an eye out for athletes who have recently had trouble at home or with the police, who are not getting along with teammates, or who seem withdrawn or overly aggressive. Also be aware of athletes whose parents never miss a practice or game and seem too eager for their child's success. All of these situations could set the stage for an injury. Appropriate intervention, whether it be a friendly chat with the athlete or parent or referral to the appropriate professional, can have valuable long-term benefits. It is always better to prevent a problem than to treat it after it has occurred.

Conclusion

Coaches and trainers should **know their athletes**—not just names but who their parents, brothers, and sisters are, whether they have been injured previously and how they reacted, their personality types, and their ability to interact with other people. Try to gain your athletes' trust. Athletes need to know that you have their best interests in mind and will be their advocate. Do not hesitate to get the advice of the team physician or to refer difficult problems to a professional.

Peter R. Coleman

27

Drug Abuse and the Athlete

In recent years, drug and alcohol abuse have become a common problem in athletics. Both mind-altering drugs and drugs that enhance performance are being utilized by athletes. These substances are becoming more widely available and, unfortunately, the pressure to be a user is increasing.

This chapter describes some of the substances currently being used and their dangers and offers suggestions on what to do if you suspect one of your athletes of substance abuse.

Steroids

There are different types of steroidal drugs. One type, **cortisone**, is used to treat skin conditions and can be injected into joints to relieve arthritic inflammation. This is not the type of steroid that is abused. Many athletes, however, take **anabolic steroids**, which increase muscle mass and strength if the athlete continues to lift weights aggressively. The side effects of these drugs are numerous. The athlete becomes more aggressive and irritable. Acne becomes worse, blood pressure increases, and sex drive decreases. Long-term side effects are liver damage, liver cancer, and heart attacks.

One survey found that 5 percent of high school students were using anabolic steroids. Not all of these were athletes, but they all wanted to improve their body size and strength—some to increase performance and others to enhance their image.

Be suspicious of any athlete who displays tremendous and rapid increases in bulk and strength, out of proportion to his or her peers. Remember that the steroid user is likely to be more aggressive and has probably had a personality change in addition to the physical change.

Educate your athletes about steroids. Although the drugs may allow them to increase their body size and strength, no one has documented any increase in performance attributable to steroids. Good, conscientious weight training will give athletes all they need to increase their performance and gain a competitive edge.

The bad effects of steroids have already been mentioned. Make sure the athletes are aware of them. Steroids are illegal and dangerous, and they do not improve performance.

Speed

Amphetamines, also called "speed" or "uppers," have been in use since 1950. They are not as common now but are still abused by some who want to get a quick lift. Athletes who use speed think that it will improve their performance. There is some evidence that it may help runners and swimmers increase their performance by 1 to 4 percent, but there is even more evidence that performance will decrease.

The drug raises heart rate and blood pressure, increases alertness, decreases fatigue, and gives the user more energy, but it also causes shakiness of the hands, uncontrolled aggression, and sometimes confusion, paranoia, and hallucinations. The effect of the drug lasts from four to ten hours and is followed by a prolonged and intense feeling of extreme fatigue.

Deaths from amphetamine use have been reported, and the drug is both physically and psychologically addicting. Mood swings and dramatic changes in performance are signals that you should note. The best treatment is to educate your athletes about the dangers of speed.

Marijuana

"Pot," "reefers," "dope," "weed," and "grass" are some of the common street names for marijuana, a widely used and abused drug. The average user is between sixteen and twenty-five years of age. It is estimated that 2 percent of high school and college students use the drug at least once a week.

When smoked, marijuana causes a mild feeling of euphoria with a slight distortion of consciousness and reality. The user feels relaxed and free of worry and has an increased appetite. But the drug also impairs insight and judgment and may cause the user to feel that people are against him or her.

The smoke from marijuana is more damaging to the lungs than regular cigarette smoke, and use of the drug by pregnant women may cause birth defects. But the most devastating effect of marijuana use is loss of motivation and stagnation of emotional growth.

Athletes who use marijuana are usually poor performers. You should suspect use of the drug if both performance and the desire to achieve begin to decrease.

Cocaine

Cocaine has become a widely abused drug today. A 1985 survey showed that 40 percent of high school seniors had tried it. Cocaine is the most addicting of all drugs. Once hooked, the user will do anything to obtain the drug. In fact, experimental animals that become addicted prefer cocaine to food and sleep.

Cocaine can be injected, smoked, or snorted through the nose. Cocaine rapidly infuses the user with a strong sense of power and control and a feeling of invincibility.

It imparts a rush of euphoria that lasts about twenty minutes. This is followed by severe depression and craving for a return to the euphoric state. Paranoia, confusion, and abnormal heart rhythms are possible side effects, and deaths from heart attacks have occurred. Fatalities have also resulted from performing dangerous acts under the influence of the drug.

It takes money to support a cocaine habit, so some users may choose to work rather than to play sports, thereby decreasing the number of athletes who use cocaine. Education of your athletes—especially of those gifted athletes who may, in the future, be able to earn money because of their athletic abilities—is the most important way to prevent cocaine use.

Alcohol

"Booze" is the most widely abused substance in society. About 60 percent of adults drink alcohol. The average age at which a person takes his or her first drink is twelve to fifteen years of age. Alcohol is a chemical depressant that reduces inhibitions, encourages relaxation, and makes people feel more lively, happy, and sociable. Just one drink, though, begins to depress function and judgment. As one continues to drink, one loses the ability to think clearly and make coordinated movements. Alcohol abuse damages the liver, brain, pancreas, bone marrow, nerves, and heart.

In young people, occasional alcohol use has been shown to cause chemical changes in the liver and to reduce muscle strength and coordination. For these reasons, it is inadvisable for athletes to use alcohol in any form because it will decrease performance. The negative effects may last for four to five days following consumption of alcohol.

Dealing with Alcohol and Drug Abuse

The symptoms and patterns exhibited by athletes with drug abuse problems are subtle and difficult to detect in their early stages. The symptoms do not manifest themselves all at once and are frequently covered up or brushed aside. Most athletes will deny having a problem, and we tend to abet them in that denial. It is not unusual to think that a particular athlete is just having a run of bad luck or is not having a good day.

Lack of control is the hallmark of drug and alcohol abuse. Difficulty in completing assignments, a decrease in reliability, problems with relationships, and poor school performance can all signal athletes' loss of ability to control their lives. Some other warning signs are frequent talk and jokes about getting high or driving at excessive speeds, exaggerated mood swings, and a loss of temper in response to any type of criticism.

If you suspect one of your athletes of substance abuse, check out your suspicions with your fellow coaches and some of the athlete's other teachers. If there is a problem, you will not be the only one to notice that something is different. The next step is to check things out with the athlete's family. They usually will welcome your interest because frequently they are already aware there is a problem and are frustrated about how to deal with it. Your subsequent actions will vary depending on school policy and your level of comfort in tackling the problem. Don't discount the impact you can have on your athletes, who have a tremendous amount of respect for you.

Some coaches and trainers become angry when they uncover an abuse problem and just want to get rid of the athlete. You should always keep in mind that, although the athlete may become ineligible for the team because of the abuse, he or she still needs support to overcome the problem. Remember that adolescence is a time of great turmoil, and the coaches and team may be the main source of support for the athlete.

The best treatment for alcohol and drug abuse is prevention, and the primary means of prevention are education and the adoption of appropriate role models. Ask your team physicians or other knowledgeable individuals to discuss the dangers of drug and alcohol use and abuse with your team. Do this more than once a year so your athletes know it is important.

Be a role model. Athletes should never smell alcohol on the breath of any coach, trainer, physician, or any other adult associated with the team. Drinking and recreational drug use should never be mentioned in a joking or matter-of-fact manner. Don't be afraid to express your views about how dangerous drugs and alcohol can be. Saying nothing is sometimes considered the same as condoning the act.

Section 4

Administrative
Issues

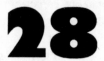

The Training Room

More and more high schools are finding that sports medicine is critical to the success of their entire athletic program. Establishing a quality training facility is a major part of developing a comprehensive sports medicine program at the high school level. In order for the training room to serve the school in the most effective manner, several important issues must be decided before opening such a facility. These issues include: (1) size and composition of the training room staff; (2) which school needs the facility will serve (e.g., physical education classes, intramurals, classroom accidents, etc.); and (3) the maximum number of students the facility will need to accommodate during peak hours. These considerations should direct the ultimate design of the training room.

Without a doubt, the most important asset to a training room is a certified athletic trainer. Without such a person, an abundance of supplies, training kits, and high-tech equipment cannot make a sports medicine program. The specific responsibilities of athletic trainers vary from school to school, depending on whether they are certified through the National Athlete Trainers Association (NATA). However, any trainer will have certain responsibilities regardless of certification. These include the administration of first aid and cardiopulmonary resuscitation (CPR), taping, bandaging, wrapping and protecting injuries, and supervising the athletic training facility.

A training room should have several characteristics in order to achieve optimal function.

The room should be located in or near the locker rooms and should be accessible to both male and female athletes. It should have electricity and water hookups (hot and cold), proper lighting, and adequate ventilation. The minimum space necessary for a training room is 15' × 30' (450 square feet). This allows room for a taping table, a treatment table, a sink, counter space, and such basic equipment as a refrigerator, ice machine, and whirlpool.

The appropriate size of the room depends on the number of athletes that will need to be accommodated. One taping table can hold 20 people and requires approximately 100 square feet of space. This estimate includes the table size, the working area, and the associated counter and storage space. To determine how many tables you need, divide the number of athletes the area is to serve by 20, then multiply the result by 100; the final total is the approximate number of square feet needed for your training room.

Treatment tables and taping tables can be built by any high school shop or woodworking class. Treatment tables should measure 30" high, 2' wide, and 6'–7' long. They are usually covered with foam and a vinyl upholstery. Taping tables are roughly half the length of treatment tables.

Another important factor in setting up the training room is the arrangement of equipment. Ideally the hydrotherapy equipment (refrigerator, ice machine, and whirlpool) should be in a separate area of the training room, both to localize the water connections and to cut down on the noise. If space is limited, isolate this equipment in one corner of the room. Other than the items already mentioned, a training room needs a desk, a chair, a file cabinet, and a telephone. Set aside some space for locking up such items as medications, supplies, or physician's equipment.

Floors should be concrete, covered with a nonslip surface that is easily cleaned. Training rooms are frequently entered directly from muddy fields and grassy trails, and a floor that is simple and easy to maintain is a necessity. The walls should be light colored to help create an "antiseptic" look, all electric outlets should be grounded, and the doors should be wide enough to accommodate a stretcher.

An adequately supplied training room always has the following on hand: athletic tape, elastic bandages, ankle wraps, Band-Aids, gauze pads, alcohol, hydrogen peroxide, antibacterial ointments, moleskin, adhesive foam and felt, external analgesics, lubricants, plastic bags, pa-

per cups, thermometer, blood pressure cuff, stethoscope, scissors, tape cutters, crutches, arm slings, knee immobilizers, cervical collars, finger splints, coolers, and training kits. Ordinarily the athletic trainer monitors the supplies in the training room.

Another critical aspect of a well-run training room is an efficient record-keeping system. Preparticipation physical exams, insurance forms, daily treatment logs, injury report forms, emergency information cards, and physician's reports and recommendations must all be kept current and available. Examples of these forms can be obtained from The Sports Medicine Foundation of America, Inc., 615 Peachtree Street, N.E., Suite 1100, Atlanta, Georgia.

An adequate training facility, staffed by a qualified athletic trainer, is a major advantage for any athletic program. However, the training facility needs to be set up with careful planning and foresight if it is to be truly beneficial.

Robbie H. Lester

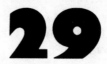

Teacher Athletic Trainers

It would be ideal if every school had an athletic trainer certified by the National Athletic Trainers Association. This should be our goal, but until that goal is achieved, we need interim solutions. One such solution is the Teacher Athletic Trainer program being utilized in the state of North Carolina. This program has helped reduce the number of high school athletes who are injured and reinjured. The Teacher Athletic Trainer (TAT) is a teacher who has developed some minimal skills as a trainer through the unique program described in this chapter.

Purpose of the Teacher Athletic Trainer

A TAT is primarily concerned with the prevention, emergency treatment, and rehabilitation of sports injuries and the provision of paramedical lifesaving services such as first aid and cardiopulmonary resuscitation (CPR) to students participating in any school activity. TATs are employed by local schools to coordinate the sports medicine program and provide these services. The TAT must be committed to the safety of students who participate in sports and other school activities and must work to prevent all deaths and disabling injuries

as well as to reduce the total incidence of injuries and reinjuries. These responsibilities are fulfilled by working with the medical resources available in the local community and by developing a medical delivery system to benefit the students.

The varied responsibilities of the TAT require a versatile individual. The most important of these obligations is the classroom instruction for which the teacher is chiefly employed. Athletic training duties are carried out in addition to teaching commitments and should be compensated as extracurricular activities. A TAT is responsible for establishing working relationships with the principal, the athletic director, and the team or consulting physician as well as with the students.

Specific training is required for the TAT to provide quality athletic training services. At the present time, four basic courses represent the minimum educational requirements established by the North Carolina State Board of Education. These are Cardiopulmonary Resuscitation (CPR), Standard First Aid, Basic Athletic Training, and Advanced Athletic Training. These courses fulfill minimal requirements and **do not** represent certification. First aid and CPR courses are available through local community service agencies. Basic and advanced athletic training are available through regional courses sponsored by the Sports Medicine Program of the North Carolina Department of Public Instruction or through the North Carolina Athletic Trainers Association Clinic, which is conducted annually in conjunction with the North Carolina Coaches Association Clinic and East/West All-Star Games in Greensboro.

Justification for Teacher Athletic Trainers

Statistics indicate that schools employing TATs have lower rates of injury and reinjury than those with no TATs. The schools that lack TATs have an average injury rate of 50 percent and a reinjury rate of 71 percent, whereas schools that employ TATs have an injury rate of 22 percent and a reinjury rate of 11 percent. Statistics also indicate that the higher the TAT's level of education and training in sports medicine, the lower the injury rate. Where the athletic trainer is certified by the National Athletic Trainers Association (NATA), the reinjury rate is 3 percent.

Thanks to the evidence of dramatic reductions in injuries and reinjuries demonstrated by these statistical studies, in 1979 the North Carolina General Assembly ratified House Bill 618, "An Act to Provide Sports Medicine and Emergency Life Saving Services to Students in the Public Schools." So important did the legislators consider the need for teacher athletic trainers that their bill required the State Board of Education to develop plans to place a TAT in every high school. The board's Basic Education Program states that "all high schools are required to employ a TAT who is qualified to provide sports medicine to students injured in interscholastic athletics and provide paramedical services to those students and/or teachers injured during regular school hours."

Employment of Teacher Athletic Trainers

The Sports Medicine Program of the State Department of Public Instruction assists schools in employing and/or training TATs. The options available for employment of TATs are as follows:

• A school may hire a teacher who already has sports medicine and paramedical skills, preferably an athletic trainer certified according to NATA standards. Al-

though North Carolina does not have a certification standard, NATA certification represents the highest level of expertise attainable by an athletic trainer. NATA-certified athletic trainers have met stringent educational requirements and have passed a national certification exam, which consists of a written section as well as an oral practical section.

• A school may select a current faculty member who is interested in sports and is willing to learn as much as possible about sports medicine. This faculty member can be educated through staff development programs. The State Board of Education has approved the four courses mentioned earlier as the minimum requirements to qualify a teacher as an athletic trainer.

The Department of Public Instruction encourages TATs to continue their education in sports medicine beyond the minimum requirements for the program. TATs are also encouraged to complete the Instructor's Level courses in first aid and CPR so that they can provide greater service to their schools by instructing coaches and faculty members in these lifesaving skills and techniques.

Athletic Injury Reports and Records

Record keeping is a vital part of any sports medicine program. It is very important that the TAT keep accurate and up-to-date records of injuries to student athletes. These records should include logs of daily treatments as well as notations of physician referrals. A note should be made each time an athlete is treated by the TAT or evaluated by a physician and each time an athlete's activity is restricted by the TAT or the physician. Physician release forms, which indicate permission for an athlete to return to activity, should always be on file.

Staff and Assistants of Teacher Athletic Trainers

A TAT's job is very demanding; therefore, consideration should be given to the development of a staff of student trainers. With proper training and education in sports medicine, these students can provide a valuable service to the high school athletic program. The TAT can also educate coaches in the management of sports-related injuries. These coaches will be able to provide emergency services until the athlete can be seen by the TAT and/or physician. It is important that all coaches recognize common injuries and know how to treat them. A TAT is responsible for establishing guidelines to ensure that all sports will be covered by coaches, physicians, and/or student assistants.

Responsibilities of Teacher Athletic Trainers

The overall responsibilities of the TAT may vary from one school to another. The list of **recommended** responsibilities given below should be reviewed by each TAT and the school administration to determine the specific duties of the TAT at the school to which he or she is assigned.

Administrative Responsibilities

• Coordinate sports medicine services for the entire school sports system.
• Serve as liaison between athletes, parents, the coach, and the consulting physician in matters relating to the prevention, care, and management of athletic injuries.
• Arrange for a team physician.
• Arrange preparticipation medical examinations by a medical doctor for all student athletes.
• Coordinate physician coverage for practice sessions and events in contact sports.
• Maintain a file on the medical history of all student athletes, including daily injury records, daily treatment records, and physician referral and release records.
• Process all insurance forms for medical fees and charges concerning sports-related injuries to student athletes.
• Maintain personal records on each student athlete in order to facilitate communications with parents or guardians regarding serious injuries.
• Plan and develop an athletic training area (room) to meet the needs of student athletes.
• Budget for and purchase supplies and equipment for the training room.
• Coordinate policies and procedures for the training room with coaches and school administrators.
• Coordinate sports medicine services for the team(s) at away games.
• Assist visiting teams with any necessary medical help when requested.

Supervisory, Advisory, and Instructional Services

• Supervise and maintain the athletic training facility.
• Supervise the dressing areas and shower facilities to ensure the maintenance of good hygiene, sanitation, and safety.
• Supervise the student trainer staff and any volunteers involved in sports medicine activities.
• Advise and counsel the coaching staff and athletic administration regarding the safety factors of the athletic program's equipment and facilities.
• Advise and counsel athletes and parents about nutrition and other health needs.
• Advise and counsel athletes and parents about emergency treatment that may be needed for injuries.
• Provide instruction in CPR and first aid to the coaching staff and other teachers.

Prevention of Injuries

• Develop fitness screening programs for student athletes who previously have been approved by a physician for participation in school sports.
• Advise students and coaches on planning and implementing preseason and off-season conditioning programs involving strength, flexibility, endurance, power, agility, and coordination of specific body parts for specific sports.
• Advise and supervise student athletes and coaches in prepractice flexibility and warm-up drills.
• Advise and supervise the selection, fitting, and maintenance of protective equipment.
• Routinely inspect protective equipment.
• Plan for and supervise the use of mouth protection devices.
• Coordinate the inspection of athletic playing facilities.
• Coordinate with coaches the necessary water breaks and rest periods for students practicing and playing in hot, humid weather.
• Monitor players for fatigue and for excessive weight gains and/or losses.
• Supervise dietary supplementation plans (added salt, potassium, iron, calcium, vitamins, etc.) relevant to athletic participation.
• Coordinate and implement in-service instructional programs for coaches regarding the prevention and management of injuries.
• Apply such techniques and devices as strapping, ban-

daging, braces, or special protective equipment designed to prevent or protect athletic injuries.

• Be able to design and build any special injury protection pads or devices needed to enable injured athletes to participate without subjecting the athlete to further injury.

Emergency Treatment of Injuries

• Plan and organize—with administrators, athletic directors, coaches, and team physicians—emergency procedures for athletes and other students injured in school activities, including the availability of emergency rescue teams for games and high-risk practice sessions.

• Plan and arrange with host schools the availability of emergency medical services for away games.

• Ensure the availability of necessary emergency equipment and coordinate the use of proper first aid techniques involving that equipment.

• Evaluate injuries according to location and severity and arrange appropriate transportation for the injured student.

• Provide care and management of minor injuries not requiring the services of a physician.

• Observe injured athletes for signs and symptoms of conditions that may require physician referral.

• Refer to a physician any injuries requiring additional medical attention.

• Provide information to assist the physician in evaluating and/or diagnosing injuries.

• Serve as liaison between the physician and injured athletes and parents in matters concerning the diagnosis, status, and progress of an injury.

• Serve as liaison between the physician and coaching staff.

Post-Injury Care

• Provide post-injury care as prescribed by the consulting physician.

• Supervise the activities of injured student athletes who are unable to participate in practice or whose participation has been restricted.

• Plan and organize selected exercises and drills to maintain the conditioning level of injured athletes in order to facilitate their return to participation.

• Keep coaches informed about the progress of injured athletes and the degree to which these students may participate in practice sessions.

• Provide reports to the physician on the progress of an injured athlete who is under that physician's care.

• Advise the coaches, as directed by the consulting physician, of when an athlete may practice following injury or illness.

• Implement reconditioning programs recommended by the consulting physician.

Provision of Paramedical Services

• Develop and coordinate an emergency care plan for students injured in the school at which the TAT is employed.

• Be on call during the school day to provide emergency paramedical services to students participating in school activities.

• Provide first aid and CPR instruction to faculty and students.

Continued Professional Development

• Complete the minimum education requirements approved by the North Carolina Board of Education.

• Maintain current certification in first aid and CPR.

• Maintain professional growth through membership and participation in the National Athletic Trainers Association and through the clinics and workshops sponsored by the Sports Medicine Program of the State Department of Public Instruction.

Edward J. Shahady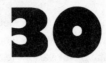

Preparticipation Evaluations

Before they participate in any sport, athletes should always have a physical exam performed by a licensed physician. Preparticipation exams have four specific goals:

1. To determine who can and who cannot participate
2. To discover medical problems that could affect participation
3 .To discover medical problems that predispose an athlete to injury
4. To provide counseling and establish a physician-athlete relationship

The History

It is important to obtain an inclusive medical history from each athlete. The form currently used by most high schools is inadequate because it does not solicit enough information to achieve all the goals of the exam. The sample form at the end of this chapter provides an example of a more inclusive history form.

A good medical history form should cover the following crucial points:

• **Family history**, especially the sudden death of a close relative under age forty-five, which may indicate an inherited heart problem
• **Medical problems** that could be influenced by ex-

ercise, such as diabetes, asthma, epilepsy, allergies, and skin infections
• **Heart trouble**, which can be signalled by the presence of chest pain or dizziness brought on by exercise
• **Problems that predispose an athlete to injury**, for example a prior concussion, which increases by seven times the athlete's chances of sustaining another concussion, or prior knee and ankle injuries, which double the chances of reinjury
• **Use of medication**, prior limitation of sports participation, and concern about injuries

The Physical

Several studies have shown that the usual preparticipation physical exam is inadequate in some areas, especially the orthopedic portion, whereas other parts of the exam are overemphasized. These studies stress that every physical should include blood-pressure testing, heart exam, orthopedic exam, and urine testing, because these are the areas that produced findings relevant to athletic participation.

The rest of the physical exam is of no value if the history reveals no positive answers.

Studies have also stressed that the physicals should be conducted by physicians who have an interest in sports medicine and who enjoy doing these exams. Too many times the physicians are too busy and are basically uninterested in their task.

177

Place of the Exam

Examinations can be performed in the physician's office or at the school. Exams in which the athletes go from station to station for various tests are acceptable as long as there is a private place in which the exam is completed by one person who reviews the history and talks to the athlete.

The preparticipation exam is the only health exam that most adolescents receive during high school or junior high. For this reason, the occasion provides an ideal opportunity for the physician to counsel athletes about drug and alcohol abuse, tobacco, and sexually transmitted diseases.

Determining Who Is in Shape

An athlete's physical condition can be determined by measuring the level of cardiovascular conditioning. Injuries, tolerance to heat, and overall athletic performance are all influenced by this conditioning. Athletes who are not in shape must be watched more closely.

The Cooper test, also called the twelve-minute run, is a simple but very effective way to test conditioning. Use the track at your school (on a standard track, each lap is equal to a quarter of a mile). Have the athletes run for twelve minutes and see how many laps they can complete in that time. Use the following table to gauge who is in shape:

Condition	Laps	Miles
Excellent	7–8	1.75–2 miles
Good	6–7	1.5–1.75 miles
Fair	5–6	1.25–1.5 miles
Poor	4–5	1–1.25 miles

For the test, have the athletes dress according to the weather (e.g., light clothing for warm days). Encourage athletes to go at a pace that does not make them sick, but be sure that the trainer is available to deal with any sickness that does occur.

Tests for flexibility and body fat content can also be part of the exam, but current research does not seem to indicate that these factors help in predicting injuries.

Health Questionnaire
for Athletic Competition

Student's name _____

Birthdate _____

Grade _____

Parent(s) name _____

Address _____

Home phone _____

Emergency phone(s) _____

Family physician _____

Family Medical History

	Y	N
Diabetes (high sugar in blood)	❏	❏
Allergies (hay fever or asthma)	❏	❏
Migraine headaches (severe and long-lasting headaches)	❏	❏
Heart trouble	❏	❏
High blood pressure	❏	❏
Sudden death (under age 45)	❏	❏

Personal Medical History

Brain concussion (head injury)	❏	❏
Tendency to lose consciousness (faint)	❏	❏
Skull fracture	❏	❏
Convulsions or epilepsy (seizures)	❏	❏
Neck injury	❏	❏
Very poor (impaired) vision in one eye	❏	❏
Temporary loss of vision	❏	❏
Glasses or contact lenses	❏	❏
Hearing loss	❏	❏
Perforated eardrum	❏	❏
Discharge from an ear (recurrent ear infections)	❏	❏
Sinus infections	❏	❏
Broken nose	❏	❏
Dental plate (one or more false teeth)	❏	❏
Braces on teeth (teeth straightened)	❏	❏
Back injury or frequent backaches	❏	❏
Knee injury (sprain) or recurrent pain in knee	❏	❏

	Y	N
Ankle injury (sprain) or recurrent pain in ankle	❏	❏
Trouble in any other joints	❏	❏
Bone infection	❏	❏
Bone fracture (broken bone)	❏	❏
Joint dislocation	❏	❏
Foot problems	❏	❏
Heart trouble or murmer	❏	❏
High blood pressure	❏	❏
Persistent cough	❏	❏
Chest pain while exercising	❏	❏
Dizziness or faintness while exercising	❏	❏
Diabetes (high sugar in blood or urine)	❏	❏
Tendency to bleed or bruise easily	❏	❏
Anemia ("tired" blood)	❏	❏
Weight problem (under- or overweight)	❏	❏
Asthma (wheezing)	❏	❏
Hay Fever	❏	❏
Abnormal or allergic reaction to bee sting	❏	❏
Abnormal or allergic reaction to medicine	❏	❏
Hives or rash	❏	❏
Fungus infection	❏	❏
Athlete's foot	❏	❏
Recurrent boils	❏	❏
Hernia or rupture	❏	❏
Kidney problems	❏	❏
Loss of function or absence of testicle(s)	❏	❏

Please Answer the Following:

1. Do you take any medicine regularly? _____
If yes, name: _____

2. Do you take medicine for emergency use? _____
If yes, name: _____

3. Have you ever been told to give up sports or limit athletic activity because of a health problem? _____

4. Do you have a health or injury problem about which you want to talk to a doctor? _____

5. Are you, or have you ever been, a tobacco smoker? _____

J. Thomas Newton

Choosing a
Team Physician

A quality sports medicine staff is a necessity for high school athletic programs, and a qualified team physician should figure prominently on that staff. Selecting the team physician is perhaps the most important step in assembling a school's or a team's sports medicine staff. Several aspects of the doctor-trainer-coach-athlete interrelationship should be considered in choosing this physician.

One essential characteristic of any team physician is a genuine interest in athletics and athletic events. The ideal candidate actively participates in some sport, and that participation provides a basic understanding of an athlete's experiences. In addition the team physician should have a true interest in the development of young athletes. He or she should be able to communicate well with both athletes and parents. A local family practitioner would be uniquely qualified, having been trained to treat all members of a family. This physician may already have an established rapport with some athletes and their parents, a connection that would facilitate communication and strengthen trust in the doctor-athlete-parent relationship.

Doctors who are new to an area also make good candidates for team physicians because the position gives them an opportunity to meet the community and build a new practice. Many physicians feel an obligation to be involved with their communities, and being a team physician helps them fulfill this obligation.

The team physician also should be able to treat ill-

nesses other than those strictly related to bones, joints, and muscles, because a significant proportion of medical problems in athletes are unrelated to those areas. These other medical problems may affect an athlete's ability to perform on a given day or in a given event. A physician who is trained to deal with all forms of illnesses is an ideal choice for the role of team physician, particularly if he or she continues to keep up with sports medicine issues through continuing education opportunities.

A team physician must work with the school officials, staff, and athletes to ensure adequate preparticipation screening for all athletes. In addition, the exam process should include the participation of other qualified, interested physicians in performing the exams as well as in reviewing the results. The team physician arranges follow-up care for any problems discovered during the exam.

The team physician's level of involvement in practices, games, and matches depends on the demands of his or her individual practice. Most doctors find it difficult to attend practice sessions but should be able to attend games. Arrangements should be made that will enable trainers and coaches to contact the team physician easily. Perhaps certain times of the day or week can be set aside to discuss problems with athletes, by phone or in person. The physician's office staff should be alerted to the needs of young athletes and instructed to arrange quick and easy access to the physician. Some team physicians arrange special clinics for the athletes, for example, each Saturday morning after Friday evening football games.

A team physician who is committed to athletics and to high school athletes, who has a broad-based knowl-edge of medical illnesses as well as orthopedic injuries, and who can relate well to coaches, trainers, and the athletes' families is a vital part of a successful sports medicine team.

Richard L. Knox

The Coach's Role in Preventing Injuries and Caring for Injured Athletes

Coaches of high school athletic teams have numerous responsibilities in caring for the health of their athletes. This chapter provides guidelines designed to help coaches organize a comprehensive program that will provide for the health needs of athletes before, during, and after injury.

• Secure the services of a trained individual, such as a team doctor, certified athletic trainer, or student trainer, to handle injuries. The coach should work with this individual to oversee an athlete's treatment, rehabilitation, and return to activity. In the event of serious injury or illness, the final decision regarding an athlete's return should rest with the team doctor, in consultation with the coach.

• Develop a form for each sport stating the risks inherent to that particular sport, potential injuries, and guidelines for the prevention and treatment of those injuries. Each form should include a statement of consent to be read and signed by both the athlete and his or her parents. Keep the signed statements on file with the athlete's medical history for quick reference in case of an emergency.

• Develop a complete emergency plan for managing on- or off-field emergencies that covers all details, such as transportation to the nearest medical facility.

• Develop a plan for diagnosing nonemergency injuries. One such plan, developed by a certified trainer, required all injured athletes to report injuries immediately following the event. The next morning the athletes were to get up at 9:00 A.M., check for any previously undetected injuries, and report immediately to the trainer for treatment. Awareness of an injury is as important as treatment, because one cannot treat an injury until it has been diagnosed.

• Supervise all activities. Coaches should always be on the scene when drills are taking place. A coach's presence may not prevent injuries, but it can give the coach firsthand knowledge of how an injury occurred as well as the opportunity to provide immediate assistance if necessary.

• Complete an injury report each time an athlete is injured and keep it on file along with the athlete's other records. Encourage injured athletes to see their family physicians. In the case of a serious injury, notify the parents as soon as possible.

• Outline the practice schedule, noting the specific purposes of various drills and how they are taught. Do not assume that your athletes already have all the necessary skills. Be thorough in teaching basic skills, as proper techniques lead to safer participation in the sport.

• Emphasize good conditioning as another important way of preventing injuries. Base conditioning exercises on the specific requirements of the sport. Have the athletes start out slowly and advance as their levels of conditioning improve.

• Make sure equipment and facilities are safe. Conduct regular checks to make sure equipment fits properly, particularly for football.

Caring for the health of athletes means doing everything possible to prevent injuries and to ensure adequate care should an athlete suffer injury. The development of a complete program designed to meet the full range of health needs is an essential first step.

Thomas D. Shahady

The Athlete's Perspective

The athlete's perspective on treatment is important and must not be overlooked. During my many years playing football, my primary reason for seeking treatment was so that I could play in the next game. My desire to play outweighed any other considerations, including the possibility of permanent damage. Many athletes want to play because they have trained hard, and they feel that coaches, parents, and classmates depend on them to perform. Young athletes must understand the seriousness of their particular injury and how continuing to play with an injury can endanger their ability to play in future games.

Players often fail to understand the importance of stretching exercises in preventing injuries. I remember times when our teams would rush through the stretching or would stretch half-heartedly or incorrectly. Coaches have a responsibility to constantly stress the importance of stretching and to allow adequate time to do it properly. Use of partners is essential to allow for maximum stretching, provide consistency, and encourage improvement.

Another area that coaches and trainers should stress is the importance of rehabilitation. Athletes often perceive rehabilitation as an additional and unnecessary burden. Having to go to the training room half an hour early only adds to the burden of practice itself. Trainers must emphasize the importance of rehabilitation and of following instructions for the use of whirlpool, heating pads, and taping to ensure full recovery from an injury.

Trainers who inspire confidence in their ability to treat injuries will be of the most help to players. One of the incidents I remember most vividly from my playing career was not a great tackle but an injury suffered by a player on the other team. While trailing the opposing quarterback on an option play, I watched as our defensive back tackled him from behind. The quarterback's knee was badly injured, and I remember how scared he looked. Most athletes are afraid of being injured; only the ones that can overcome that fear many times become professionals. When I realized that holding back increased my chance of injury, I played more aggressively and my play improved. Confidence in the trainer's ability goes a long way toward helping players overcome their fear of injury.

Finally, every player must be treated as an individual. Each person has a different tolerance for pain and susceptibility to injury. But players have also been known to use injuries to avoid hard practices. I remember many times when I would have liked to fall down because I felt I just couldn't keep going anymore. Trainers need to recognize when players may be at this point and encourage them to work harder. Also, starting players require different treatment than reserve players. As I prepared for my first year of college ball, I trained very hard during the off season because I wanted to start. However, after I thought I had secured a starting position, my off-season workouts grew less strenuous. Players assured of starting positions often begin preseason practice in poor shape and, consequently, may be more susceptible to injuries.

In summary, athletes tend to view the training staff simply as a means of ensuring their participation in every game. Trainers have the difficult task of helping athletes recognize the importance of adequate rehabilitation regardless of how frustrating or painful. Young athletes in particular must be made to understand the long-term implications of an injury compared with the short-term benefits of playing the next game.

Salli Benedict

34

Parent/Coach/ Trainer Relationships

Parents can play an important role in both the prevention and the treatment of athletic injuries. This chapter suggests a few practical guidelines designed to facilitate interactions between parents and athletic staff and to help avoid some common problems. Included are suggestions for communicating with parents about the health and safety of student athletes and for making the most of parental involvement.

Accessibility

The best thing you can do to enhance your relationship with your athletes' parents is to be accessible—give them your office hours and telephone numbers and let them know that their participation is welcome. Open communication among parents, trainers, and coaches can prevent or lessen many problems. Unfortunately, many parents may feel uncomfortable approaching you with their questions or concerns. One reason for this reticence may be that both athletes and parents believe that "meddling" may evoke a negative backlash against the athlete. Student athletes may also discourage their parents from contacting coaches and trainers about health or safety concerns because they feel embarrassed. It is extremely important to remind parents and students repeatedly that their concerns are important.

How to Communicate

Several methods can be used to inform parents about team policies regarding safety, injury prevention, and injury treatment. Preseason meetings that include parents, athletes, coaches, trainers, and the team physician are often highly effective. Written communications sent home with the students may be tossed out without being read (if the parents receive them at all); when such messages are necessary, try to stimulate interest by using few words and including pictures and graphs whenever possible to help communicate the meaning. You may want to have parents initial a tear-off portion of the flyer to indicate that it has been read. If some parents do not come to meetings or respond to written communications, you should follow up with a phone call.

The best kind of communication is informal: encourage booster clubs, fundraising activities, and parental involvement in awards banquets. The more you see of parents on an informal basis, the better your mutual understanding of policies and procedures will be.

What Parents Want to Know

The most important message coaches and trainers can give to parents is that everything possible is being done to safeguard the health and safety of their children. Specifically, you should always inform parents of policies and procedures regarding the following:

• Preseason screening, physical exams, and health requirements. Include the names of health professionals and trainers who are involved in the process.

• Safety measures and precautions for practices and games. Include information on protective equipment, hydration, diet, and so on.

• Injuries during practices and games. Be sure to mention which health professionals or trainers will be present and how parents will be notified if their child is injured. Parents often feel unsure about their roles, especially during games.

• Disciplinary measures for breaking team rules, particularly any procedures involving physical activity.

• How soon an injured athlete may return to participation and the roles of the family physician, team physician, trainer, student, coach, and parents in making this decision and in following recommendations.

Summary

Parents need to be reassured that coaches and trainers are protecting the safety of their children and that if an injury does occur, the team is capable of handling it in a professional manner. They want to know that a coach or trainer is always willing to talk to them about their concerns and to answer their questions.

Index

Abdomen (stomach): injuries to, 42, 44; muscles, 42, 46, 47; exercises, 49

Abductor (gluteus medius) strain, 90

Abrasions, 148

Acetabulum, 88

Acetaminophen, 19

Achilles tendinitis, 129

Achilles tendon rupture, 130

Acne, 147

Acromioclavicular ligament, 51

Acromion process, 51

Acute injuries, 3, 9; back, 43–45; knee, 100–105; lower leg, 115

Adductor muscle exercise, 97

Aerobic function, 161

Alcohol abuse, 167

Amnesia, 30, 31

Amphetamines, 166–67

Anabolic steroids, 166

Anatomical snuffbox, 72, 73, 74

Anemia, 155, 161

Ankle exercises, 14, 15, 125–27

Ankle injuries, 27; twisted ankle, 119; fracture, 119–20; sprains, 121–23, 135; peroneal tendon spasm and dislocation, 123–24; peroneal tendinitis, 124

Anorexia nervosa, 162

Anterior cruciate ligament tear, 100–102

Anterior drawer test, 101

Arm pain, 56, 58, 59

Arthritis, 74

Asians, 156

Aspirin, 19, 20, 152

Asthma, 151–52

Athletes, 185–86; common medical problems, 151–54; injury-prone, 164

Athlete's foot, 148

Atrophy, 4, 10

Back exercises, 44, 47, 48–49

Back injuries: upper-back bruises, 43; mid-back and kidney bruises, 44; acute lower-back pain, 44–45; chronic mid-back pain, 45–46; chronic low-back pain, 46–47; prevention of, 50

Back muscles, 43, 44

Bacterial infections, 147

Bennett's fracture, 80

Bicep muscles, 32

Biceps curl exercise, 70

Blacks, 144, 153, 156

Bleeding, 148; head, 29–30; internal, 42; subungual (fingernail), 87

Blisters, 149

Body fat, women, 160, 162

Body temperature, 143, 144, 154

Boils, 147

Bones: neck, 31; shoulder, 51; upper arm, 51, 56, 58, 64; elbow, 64; forearm, 64, 66, 72; wrist, 72; hand, 79; thigh, 88, 93, 99; ankle, 119; foot, 128; of women, 160–61

Bones, broken. See Fractures; Stress fractures

Boutonniere (buttonhole) finger, 83–84

Boxer's fracture, 79

Brachioradialis muscle, 32

Breasts, 161

Bruises. See Contusions

Bumps, to the head, 29, 30

Burners. See Stingers/burners

Bursa, 69

Bursitis: olecranon (elbow), 68–69; trochanteric (chronic hip pain), 90, 91–92; retrocalcaneal (heel), 131; women and, 161

Calcaneus (heel bone), 119

Calcanofibular ligament, 119, 121

Calcification, 81

Calcium intake, 144, 145

Calf muscle. See Gastrocnemius

Callouses, 149

Carbohydrate loading, 156–57

Cardiovascular conditioning, 8

Carpal bones, 72

Cartilage. See Meniscus

Cervical nerves, 31, 56

Cervical spine, 35

Cervical vertebrae, 31

Charley horse, 93

Cheerleaders, 139–42

Chest injuries: contusions, 41; broken rib, 41

Chest muscles, 41

Children, heel pain in (Sever's disease), 130–31

Chondromalacia (runner's knee), 106

Chondromalacia exercise, 112

Chronic injuries, 3; back, 45–47; hip pain, 91–92; lower leg, 115–16

Clavicle (collarbone), 51

Coaches, 183–84

Cocaine, 167

Cold treatment, 8, 9

Collarbone (clavicle), 51; fracture, 59

Collateral ligaments, knee, 99–100; tears, 103–5

Compartment syndromes, 115–16

Concussions, 29, 30–31, 177

Conjunctivitis (pinkeye), 40

Contact lenses, 40